The Science of Plant-Based Nutrition

RHIANNON LAMBERT

The
Science of
Plant-Based
Nutrition

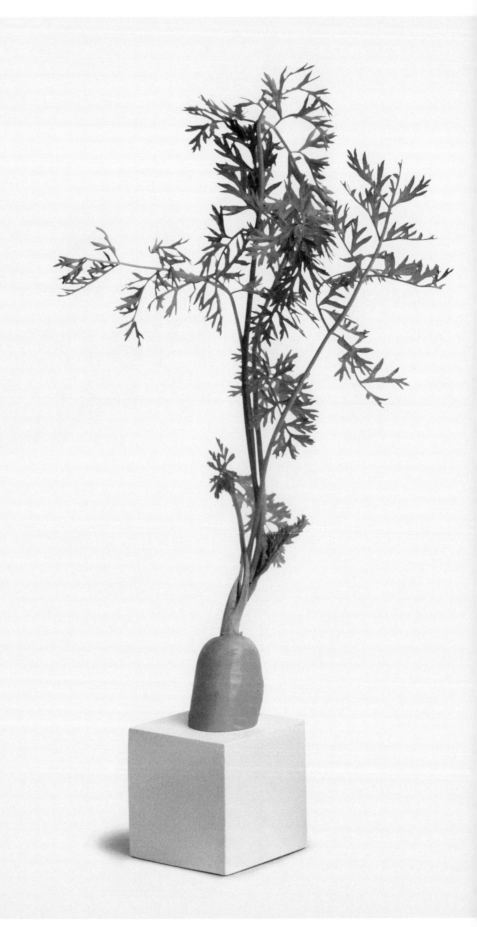

CONTENTS

INTRODUCTION

Enrolling to study nutrition at the University of Roehampton was a life-changing decision for me, and it was one that, in part, I was driven to from firsthand experience of how easily we can fall into dysfunctional relationships with food; how pressures to look a certain way can lead to a pursuit of dietary quick fixes that are a world away from a relaxed and healthy enjoyment of food.

At the age of 17, I was an aspiring soprano singer, thrust into the limelight having won Classic FM's young musician of the year. Schooled at The Royal Academy of Music and singing on stage at the likes of the Royal Albert Hall and Paris Fashion Week, I appeared to be living the most thrilling life.

But after four years suffering the pressures of the music industry, compounded by fueling myself with passing dietary fads, I looked at my career and thought: I don't want this any more. While a complete career change is rare, it is one of the best moves I ever made.

Following four grueling yet thrilling years, I obtained undergraduate and master's degrees in nutrition and started a new life as a fledgling nutritionist. Having founded Rhitrition in 2016, a private Harley Street clinic, my specialist team and I now work with individuals and leading brands to support their health and well-being. Our ethos is simple: we believe in empowering everyone to embrace a healthy way of living through the food we enjoy and the life we lead. Our bodies really are as unique as our personalities, so each of us should strive to find a way of eating that works for us individually.

It is through my experience in clinic that I have come to learn just how widespread pseudoscience is. It's everywhere, from the labels in the supermarket, on the ads that pop up in your Instagram feed, and most of all in magazines: bold statements in jargon that give the false impression they're supported by laboratory research.

This book, *The Science of Plant-Based Nutrition*, delves into the intricacies of plant-based living—from the foundations of nutrition and culinary creativity to the profound impact on personal health and the sustainability of our planet. From understanding the science behind plant-powered nutrition to navigating deficiencies and environmental concerns, *The Science of Plant-Based Nutrition* is your indispensable guide on the path to a healthier, more conscious lifestyle.

As a mother of two young boys, the welfare of our planet holds paramount importance to me. If I can play a role in facilitating positive change by guiding everyone to safely transform their diets for the betterment of both the planet and their health, it would fill me with immense pride.

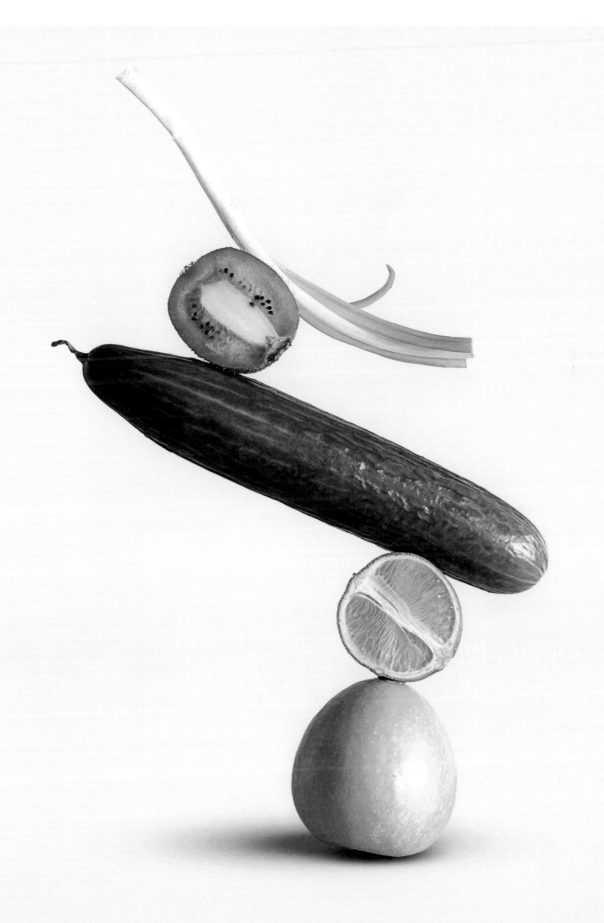

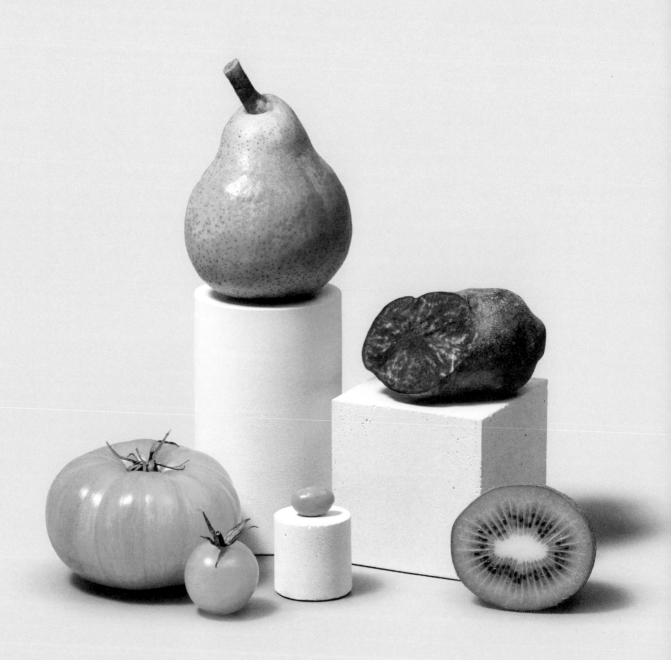

GENERAL NUTRITION

WHY IS NUTRITION SO IMPORTANT?

The food we consume contains vitamins, minerals, and nutrients that can be beneficial to our health alongside providing us with the energy needed to grow and flourish. Good nutrition is important for all areas of our health and well-being from before we are born.

WHAT IS NUTRITION?

Nutrition is the way you eat and how the food and drink that you consume delivers the nutrients you need to have a healthy body and mind. The nutrients we all require to maintain optimum health are carbohydrates, fats, fiber, protein, minerals, vitamins, and water. We should consume a healthy balance of these nutrients to grow and develop to our optimum height and stay as healthy as possible with a strong level of immunity. If you have good nutrition, you will fuel your body and brain. From conception and throughout life, nutrition provides a vital role in helping us grow optimally and stay disease-free.

Thanks to modern nutritional science, we now know a lot about the importance of good nutrition for our growth and development. If you eat a healthy, nutritionally balanced diet (see pp.26–27), it can help reduce your chances of developing serious health conditions, including diabetes, heart disease, stroke, and cancer. What you eat may also affect your brain development, mood, and mental health. Public health nutritional guidelines around the world vary from country to country and are based upon the minimum requirements needed to maintain an optimal health status and be free from disease and poor health.

THE FIRST THOUSAND DAYS

Good nutrition is important even before we are born. The health outcome of a child throughout its life is shaped by what their mother eats from the time of conception up to their second birthday (the first 1,000 days). Research in the fields of neuroscience, biology, and early childhood development provides powerful insights into how nutrition, relationships, and environments in the 1,000 days between a woman's pregnancy and a child's second birthday shape future outcomes (see pp.160–167). In countries where investment into the health and well-being of mothers and children during this crucial period is lacking, it appears that healthcare costs are higher and economic productivity lower. With a healthier and more prosperous future in mind for generations to come, several of the world's leading economists are calling for greater focus and investment in the nutrition, health, and well-being of women, babies, and toddlers during this period of growth and development.

A BRIGHTER FUTURE?

With everything we know about nutrition and the availability of whole foods, you would think that the population of the world would be in a healthier position than ever before, but sadly that is not the case. Around 37 million children are now overweight, and we are facing an obesity crisis (see pp.204–205), not only in the western world but in some lower and middle-income countries, too. This is because food systems and rising food prices are leading to more of us eating food that does not contain adequate nutrition and can result in malnourishment.

Plant-based eating and encouraging the consumption of more whole foods could be an approach that is beneficial for our nutrition and the planet. Nutrition is key to our health and happiness and everyone in the world deserves equal access to it.

Scurvy prevention

FROM THE 16TH TO THE 18TH CENTURIES, MORE THAN 2 MILLION SAILORS DIED AT SEA FROM SCURVY.

This was discovered to be due to a lack of fresh food supplies and in particular vitamin C. The Royal Navy became known as "Limeys" for carrying limes and lemons to prevent scurvy aboard their ships. Today, nutritional deficiencies are usually identified quickly and often completely eradicated in western countries, thanks to access to good nutrition and supplementation.

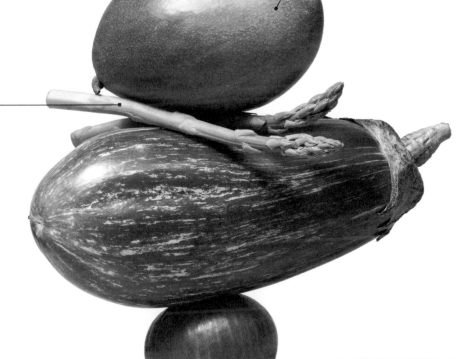

FRUIT

A FRUIT IS THE SEED-BEARING STRUCTURE IN FLOWERING PLANTS THAT IS FORMED FROM THE OVARY AFTER FLOWERING

VEGGIES

VEGETABLES ARE PARTS OF PLANTS THAT ARE CONSUMED BY HUMANS OR ANIMALS AS FOOD

HOW DO OUR BODIES PROCESS NUTRITION?

The human body is a true wonder, built perfectly to process the food we eat and draw the nutrients we require from our diets. It is far more complex than simply eating and swallowing the food we consume.

———————

The process of breaking down and absorbing the food we eat is designed to give us energy and nutrients to live and function optimally. Nutrients are then taken in the bloodstream to where they are needed in the muscles, tissues, and organs, with any waste products excreted.

MOUTH

The process of digestion begins in the mouth where food is broken down into smaller pieces by our teeth when we chew. Digestive enzymes in our saliva work to chemically break the food down further and help create a bolus—a ball of chewed up food—that is swallowed and goes through the esophagus.

ESOPHAGUS

This is a large muscular tube that extends from the epiglottis (a small flap of tissue at the back of the throat) to your stomach, transporting the food you have eaten from one end to the other. Once it reaches the stomach, the lower esophageal sphincter acts as the stomach's gateway and allows food to enter the stomach.

STOMACH

The stomach is an acidic environment where digestive enzymes and stomach acids further break down food. Muscles in the gut contract to churn and mix the food to help chemicals break it down, and the acid kills off unwanted and potentially harmful microbes found in foods. This process sends signals to the body to release a hormone called leptin, which regulates appetite by signaling that you're full. In the stomach, food is turned into chyme, a souplike consistency substance that enters the small intestine in the next phase of digestion.

SMALL INTESTINE

Food spends between 2–6 hours in the 23 ft long small intestine, being broken down by digestive enzymes so nutrients can be absorbed from the chyme into the bloodstream and to be delivered where needed to fuel and support bodily processes.

Once the nutrients have been absorbed, the remaining material moves into the large intestine.

LARGE INTESTINE

Remaining food is turned into waste in the large intestine. Undigested food can spend up to 12–30 hours here and goes from a liquid consistency to form stools, as the water is absorbed back into the body. Far from being merely a waste processor, the large intestine is home to the majority of our immune cells and a community of trillions of microbes. These gut microbiota perform many crucial processes, interacting with and supporting the immune system, hormone production, and the brain (among others) as they feed on and ferment undigested nutrients (see pp.16–17).

RECTUM AND ANUS

Finally, the semisolid waste material known as feces is excreted. This is collected in the rectum and is passed into the anus via two anal sphincters. Contraction and relaxation of the anal muscles push the stool through the sphincters and out of the anus.

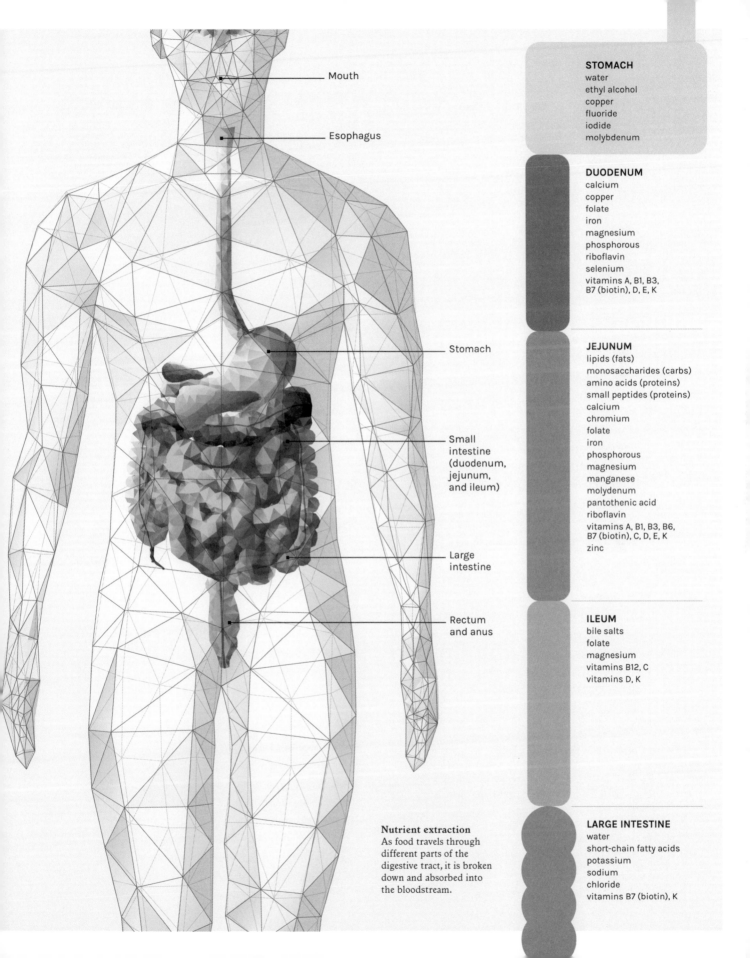

Mouth

Esophagus

Stomach

Small
intestine
(duodenum,
jejunum,
and ileum)

Large
intestine

Rectum
and anus

Nutrient extraction
As food travels through
different parts of the
digestive tract, it is broken
down and absorbed into
the bloodstream.

STOMACH
water
ethyl alcohol
copper
fluoride
iodide
molybdenum

DUODENUM
calcium
copper
folate
iron
magnesium
phosphorous
riboflavin
selenium
vitamins A, B1, B3,
B7 (biotin), D, E, K

JEJUNUM
lipids (fats)
monosaccharides (carbs)
amino acids (proteins)
small peptides (proteins)
calcium
chromium
folate
iron
phosphorous
magnesium
manganese
molydenum
pantothenic acid
riboflavin
vitamins A, B1, B3, B6,
B7 (biotin), C, D, E, K
zinc

ILEUM
bile salts
folate
magnesium
vitamins B12, C
vitamins D, K

LARGE INTESTINE
water
short-chain fatty acids
potassium
sodium
chloride
vitamins B7 (biotin), K

HOW DOES METABOLISM WORK?

Metabolism is responsible for every single chemical reaction that takes place in any living cell or organism, and it is needed to keep us alive. The food you consume provides the nutrition that gives you the energy to fuel metabolism.

What we eat provides the raw materials for metabolism, enabling it to do the essential job of creating the energy to fuel every process in the body, from energy production, growth, repair and the regulation of the cells to physical activity.

ANABOLISM AND CATABOLISM

Metabolism involves two processes working simultaneously: the building up (anabolism) and breaking down (catabolism) of molecules. Anabolic processes take place when smaller molecules called monomers are joined together to create larger molecules called polymers. For example, starch and cellulose are polymers made from the glucose monomer. Proteins are polymers of the amino acids monomers. Fats (lipids) are made from fatty acid and glycerol molecules. Because of this, fats are not polymers. Catabolic processes involve the breakdown of complex molecules into simpler ones, which causes them to release energy. This happens to the proteins, carbs, and fats that you consume in your diet. The energy is then stored and transported within cells as adenosine triphosphate (ATP).

METABOLISM AND CALORIES

Your basal metabolic rate (BMR) equates to the number of calories you need to sustain life when you are not moving. This rate varies from person to

person, and there is no fixed number of calories we need to thrive. Lifestyle changes like diet, exercise, and sleep cannot "boost" your metabolism as is often claimed, but you can choose a diet and lifestyle that supports the system, making it work more efficiently. Many factors contribute to the rate of your metabolism, including:

- Age
- Muscle mass
- Body size
- Physical activity levels

MITOCHONDRIA

Mitochondria are known as the powerhouses of a cell as they release most of the energy produced. The more energy you release, the more efficient your metabolism. Individuals who have more muscle have a higher number of mitochondria within their cells. Those who are obese tend to have a less effective metabolism (see pp.204–205).

DOES A PLANT-BASED DIET HELP OUR METABOLISM?

Some studies suggest that eating plant-based may help increase metabolism as a result of lower energy intake and weight loss. A 16-week trial of 244 Americans with a low-fat vegan diet versus a control group, which was asked to make no diet changes, found that eating a low-fat plant-based diet reduced body weight by increasing metabolism after eating and reducing energy intake. Other reviews suggest that plant-based diets help metabolic function in those with obesity and type 2 diabetes when compared to those who eat meat, but more research is emerging all the time.

Monomers
Small molecules that can join together to form polymers

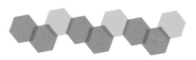

Polymers
Larger complex molecules made from smaller molecules

Energy production There are three potential energy sources from food—protein, carbs, and fats. The pathway conversion of food to cellular energy depends on what the fuel is composed of. Hormones regulate the processes of anabolism and catabolism, which work at the same time.

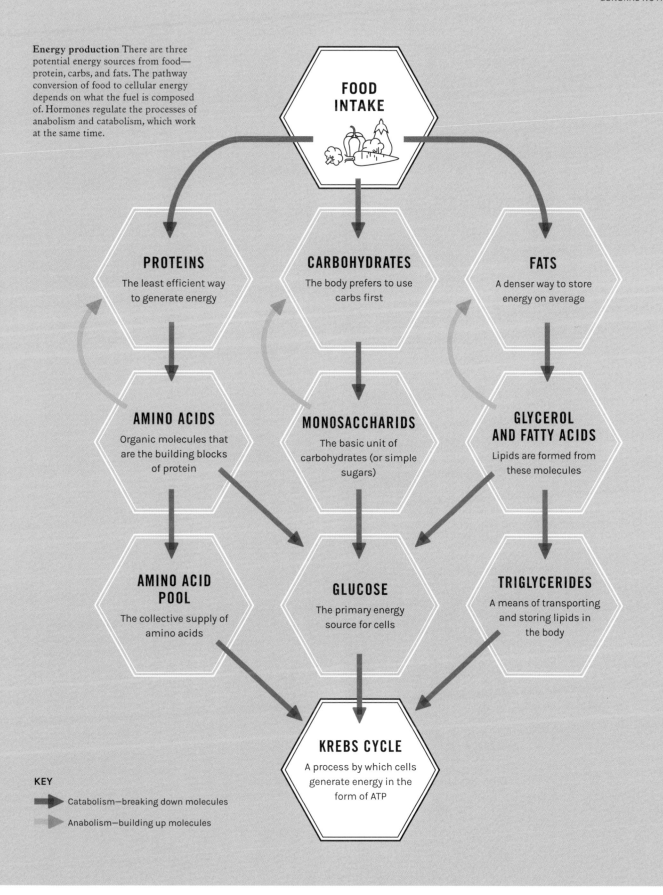

FOOD INTAKE

PROTEINS
The least efficient way to generate energy

CARBOHYDRATES
The body prefers to use carbs first

FATS
A denser way to store energy on average

AMINO ACIDS
Organic molecules that are the building blocks of protein

MONOSACCHARIDS
The basic unit of carbohydrates (or simple sugars)

GLYCEROL AND FATTY ACIDS
Lipids are formed from these molecules

AMINO ACID POOL
The collective supply of amino acids

GLUCOSE
The primary energy source for cells

TRIGLYCERIDES
A means of transporting and storing lipids in the body

KREBS CYCLE
A process by which cells generate energy in the form of ATP

KEY

→ Catabolism—breaking down molecules

→ Anabolism—building up molecules

WHAT IS MEANT BY GUT HEALTH?

The gut is a term used to describe your gastrointestinal (GI) system, the health of which is generally determined by the levels and types of bacteria in your intestinal tract. Gut health refers to the overall health of your digestive system.

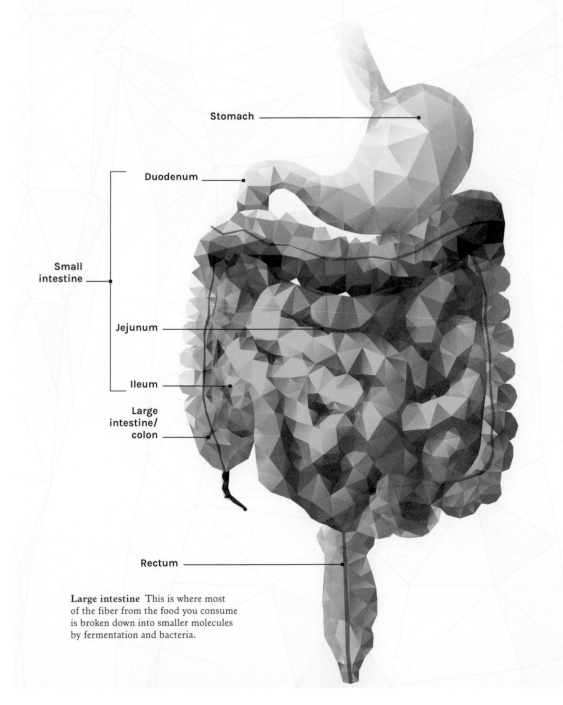

Stomach

Duodenum

Small intestine

Jejunum

Ileum

Large intestine/colon

Rectum

Large intestine This is where most of the fiber from the food you consume is broken down into smaller molecules by fermentation and bacteria.

FIVE CRITERIA FOR A HEALTHY GUT HAVE BEEN DEFINED AS FOLLOWS:

NORMAL DIGESTION, FOOD ABSORPTION, AND REGULAR BOWEL MOVEMENT

NO GASTROINTESTINAL DISEASE SUCH AS IBD, CELIAC DISEASE, REFLUX DISEASE, OR COLON CANCER

A HEALTHY FUNCTIONING INTESTINAL MICROBIOTA

GOOD IMMUNE FUNCTION

A GENERAL FEELING OF WELL-BEING AND GOOD HEALTH

Know your gut terms

In the human body, there are trillions of microorganisms. The majority of these are in the gut, where they play a vital role in our health and well-being.

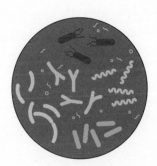

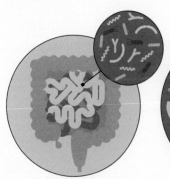

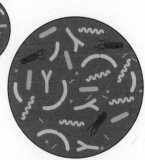

Microorganisms
Tiny living organisms, such as bacteria, viruses, or fungi.

Microbiota
A group of microorganisms in a particular location.

Microbiome
Entire genetic material of microorganisms in a specific environment.

THE MICROBIOME

"Gut health" is now synonymous with the microbiome of the large intestine but has a wider meaning, especially in clinical fields, relating to the health of the entire gastrointestinal tract. The gut microbiome consists of all the microorganisms, such as bacteria and fungi, that live in our gut. The gut influences all parts of our body, from the immune system to our digestive functions. It plays a key part in keeping our energy levels up and helping us avoid illness, so it is worth keeping it healthy.

Having a diet high in fibrous foods, found in abundance in a healthy plant-based diet, such as in nuts and whole grains, aids digestion. However, in order to digest fiber properly, we need to have the right balance of bacteria and other microorganisms in our gut. Bacteria thrives on the fiber in our diet.

The biochemical products made in our gut from foods play an important role in maintaining the normal functioning of the immune system, and producing hormones responsible for mood, hunger, and sleep regulation. The gut is also a production site for nutrients such as B vitamins.

HEALTHY GUT, HEALTHY BODY

Having a healthy gut means that the food and drink we consume day-to-day can be digested efficiently and the nutrients from them can be used to support regulating our appetite and mood. This, in turn,

helps us stay healthy and promotes well-being. Taking steps to consume foods that are helpful to our gut is a great way to keep it healthy. However, there are also foods that can harm it. Artificial sweeteners, hydrogenated fats, emulsifiers, additives, and flavorings in processed snacks can reduce the healthier gut bacteria and cause an imbalance of microorganisms in our gut. So aim to keep these foods to a minimum. Staying hydrated and taking part in regular exercise also both help the digestive system to function normally.

THE ROLE OF STRESS

Stress strongly influences our body's processes and how it functions. High levels or chronic low levels of stress can alter the microbiome, unbalancing the levels of bacteria present. Stress has also been shown to reduce the strength of the gut barrier, allowing bacteria to leak into our bodies and cause inflammation. Additionally, stress can influence the types of foods we choose and can make us go for more ultra-processed foods that are high in salt, sugar, and fat, which harm rather than support our gut health. For all these reasons, implementing stress-reducing measures is crucial for gut health. Try to include short windows of mindfulness, such as breathing exercises and meditation, throughout the day to keep stress levels lowered. Regular exercise can also help reduce your stress.

WHAT ARE COMMON PROBLEMS WITH DIGESTING FOOD?

Most of us will experience a degree of digestive discomfort at some point in our lives. In fact, 66 percent of Americans have gastrointestinal issues, and 73 percent of those aged 18–44 suffer with symptoms such as bloating, constipation, and diarrhea at least a few times a month.

———

When food is not digested properly, it can cause stomach discomfort, like bloating and abdominal pain, and lead to nutrient deficiencies and malabsorption. This results in diarrhea or constipation, weight changes, and nutritional imbalances, all of which can disrupt the gut microbiota (seepp.16–17) and affect your overall health and immune function.

The most common digestive issues are related to travel, lack of sleep, lifestyle, age, stress, and diet. If the digestive system isn't working well, it can lead to a variety of concerns from gastrointestinal discomfort, food intolerance, irregular bowel movements, and a weakened immune system. Make sure that you seek advice from your doctor if you have any concerns.

TRAVEL

Up to 50 percent of travelers experience gut health concerns on their trips. Flying in an airplane can impact our digestion because of the air pressure in the cabin itself. Any air trapped inside your gut

will expand, causing bloating and gas, in the same way as a water bottle inflating after takeoff. Your digestion is also affected by changes in time zones that disrupt your natural sleep-wake cycle (the circadian rhythm). When you are suddenly awake at a time your body is not adjusted to, this impacts your gut microbes because they are used to working at regular times. What's more, food you consume on vacation likely has different properties to your usual diet, and your gut bacteria will need new digestive enzymes to deal with this. Disruption to our normal routine can also cause problems related to processing nutrition.

AGE AND LIFESTYLE

Apart from travel and diet, the two main factors that negatively influence the health of the intestines are reduced blood flow (caused by a sedentary lifestyle) and increased pressure on the intestines, due to the compression of the intestinal organs between the hip and the diaphragm.

If you sit in one position at a desk for long periods, this can cause compression of the digestive system. Remember to get up, stretch, and move around regularly to avoid digestive issues because of this. Stress levels also impact how well our food is digested. Studies are also now looking into the impact of sedentary lifestyles on the gut microbiome, with the majority showing a negative influence from a less active lifestyle. Our digestion also naturally slows down as we age, although diet and exercise can improve matters.

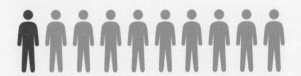

IBS GLOBAL FIGURES
It is believed that irritable bowel syndrome affects more than 1 in 10 people globally. IBS has many symptoms and can be eased through diet and exercise.

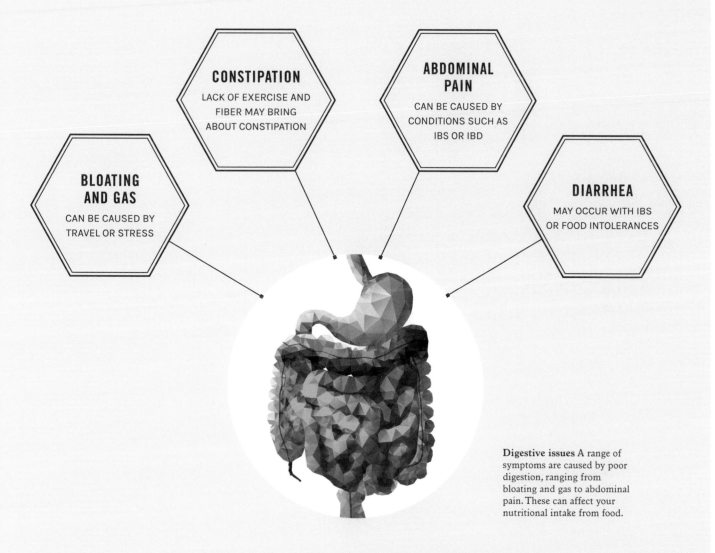

CONSTIPATION
LACK OF EXERCISE AND
FIBER MAY BRING
ABOUT CONSTIPATION

ABDOMINAL
PAIN
CAN BE CAUSED BY
CONDITIONS SUCH AS
IBS OR IBD

BLOATING
AND GAS
CAN BE CAUSED BY
TRAVEL OR STRESS

DIARRHEA
MAY OCCUR WITH IBS
OR FOOD INTOLERANCES

Digestive issues A range of
symptoms are caused by poor
digestion, ranging from
bloating and gas to abdominal
pain. These can affect your
nutritional intake from food.

IBS AND OTHER DIGESTIVE CONDITIONS

A common digestive complaint, irritable bowel
syndrome (IBS) can cause symptoms like stomach
cramps, bloating, diarrhea, and constipation.
These tend to come and go over time and can
last for days, weeks, or months. Food can pass too
quickly or too slowly, and you can have oversensitive
nerves in your gut. Stress can trigger the condition,
and a family history of IBS may enhance your
likelihood of getting it, but the cause is still
unknown and there is no cure. IBS is managed
through lifestyle and diet (see pp.82–83). Some

people also live with chronic conditions that impact
their digestion, causing severe tummy pain and
diarrhea. These include inflammatory bowel disease
(IBD) and celiac disease.

EATING DISORDERS

Anorexia and bulimia are often not thought of as a
cause of poor digestion, but they can cause damage
by weakening muscles in the gut. Other problems are
severe nausea and vomiting, esophageal erosions,
heartburn, and gastrointestinal symptoms. These
problems may be helped with appropriate treatment.

WHAT ARE MACRONUTRIENTS?

Your diet requires key components in order for your body to have enough energy and nutrition to carry out its daily tasks. The focus of these functions is largely dependent on the three macronutrients—carbohydrates, proteins, and fats.

CARBOHYDRATES

Carbohydrates are essentially sugar molecules that are broken down in the body and used as energy. Carbohydrates are often described as simple or complex, and this relates to their chemical structure. Simple carbs provide a quick burst of energy, whereas complex carbohydrates are released more slowly (see pp.94–95), often owing to their fiber content. Carbohydrates should provide around 50 percent of your total energy requirements.

PROTEIN

Protein is needed for growth and repair, is in every cell in the body, and should make up around 25 percent of our daily diet. It is made up of amino acids, both essential and nonessential. The body cannot make the nine essential amino acids itself; they need to come from our diet (see pp.92–93). Some sources of food, known as complete proteins—contain all these essential amino acids. These are mostly animal products, although some plant

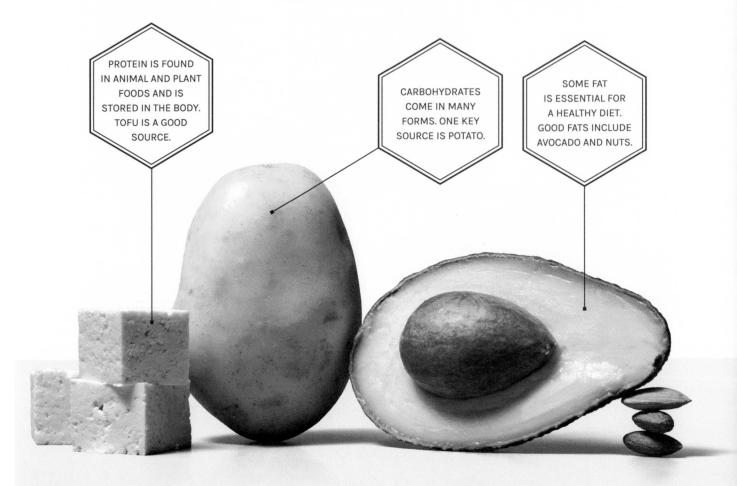

PROTEIN IS FOUND IN ANIMAL AND PLANT FOODS AND IS STORED IN THE BODY. TOFU IS A GOOD SOURCE.

CARBOHYDRATES COME IN MANY FORMS. ONE KEY SOURCE IS POTATO.

SOME FAT IS ESSENTIAL FOR A HEALTHY DIET. GOOD FATS INCLUDE AVOCADO AND NUTS.

Amino acids

Twenty types of amino acids are combined in different ways to form proteins the body needs, such as keratin for hair, hemoglobin for blood, and collagen for connective tissue.

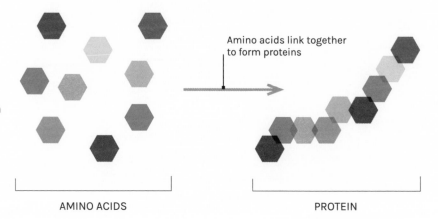

Amino acids link together to form proteins

AMINO ACIDS

PROTEIN

sources such as quinoa, soy, and hemp are essential proteins. Other plant foods are incomplete proteins and contain some of the amino acids needed on a daily basis. If you eat a varied diet across the day, you will very likely be able to get all the amino acids you require with a plant-based diet.

FAT

There are two main types of fat: saturated and unsaturated. We should aim to reduce our intake of saturated fat and eat unsaturated fat for the best health benefits.

Saturated fat is usually solid at room temperature and found mainly in animal produce, such as meat, poultry, butter, and cheese. It is also found in some plant foods, including coconut oil and palm oil.

Unsaturated fats can be monounsaturated (found in olive oils and nuts) or polyunsaturated (found in flaxseeds and chia seeds). These fats are liquid at room temperature and mostly come from plant sources such as rapeseed, olives, nuts, and seeds.

Naturally present in some dairy and meats, trans fats are also found in processed and hardened vegetable oils. Industrial trans fat or hydrogenated fat is created by adding hydrogen to oil. Lots of processed foods used to have hydrogenated fats

added to them to extend shelf life. Trans fat is harmful to our health, increasing the risk of death by 34 percent. A diet high in trans fats can raise levels of "bad" cholesterol or LDL (low-density lipoprotein) in the blood, leading to a greater risk of heart disease. Many countries have taken steps to eliminate trans fats in the manufacturing process and it is best to avoid it altogether if possible.

"Good" vs. "bad" fats

BENEFITS TO HEALTH

Monounsaturated fat: Linked to several health benefits, including reduced risk of heart disease and diabetes.

Polyunsaturated fat: One type, omega-3 fatty acids, are linked with reduced risk of neurodegenerative disease, heart disease, and diabetes.

RISKS TO HEALTH

Saturated and trans fat: Too much in the diet is linked to high cholesterol and type 2 diabetes.

WHAT ARE MICRONUTRIENTS?

Micronutrients are needed by the body in small amounts to help support the functioning of the nervous system, to support immunity, and to keep skin and hair healthy, among other things. They include vitamins and minerals.

Micronutrients are important for many reasons, including enabling the body to produce enzymes, hormones, and other substances needed for normal growth and development. Deficiencies of micronutrients can be dangerous and cause severe harm and illness. The most common deficiencies around the world are in iron, vitamin A, and iodine, particularly in children and pregnant women.

There are two types of vitamins, water soluble and fat soluble. Water-soluble vitamins are not stored in the body and if taken to excess are excreted in the urine. Fat-soluble vitamins are soluble in dietary fats and can be stored in the body. Minerals provide us with more important nutrients for our health and body.

Sources of B vitamins

There are eight B vitamins, and they play essential roles in physiological functions. They are not stored by the body, so they must be eaten regularly to stay healthy.

WATER-SOLUBLE VITAMINS:

● **Vitamin B** makes red blood cells; maintains the cardiovascular, nervous, and immune systems; and reduces fatigue by helping release energy from food.

● **Vitamin C** is an antioxidant that protects cells from damage and supports the functioning of the immune system. It plays a role in collagen production, helping with skin elasticity, and is needed to maintain healthy skin, blood vessels, and cartilage.

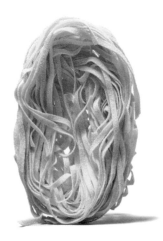

B1—THIAMINE

Plant sources
Enriched noodles, sunflower seeds, fortified cereals, whole grains, lentils

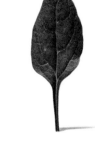

B2—RIBOFLAVIN

Plant sources
Spinach, peas, fortified cereals, mushrooms, almonds

B3—NIACIN

Plant sources
Peanuts, fortified wheat flour, whole grains, legumes

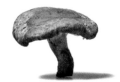

B5—PANTOTHENIC ACID

Plant sources
Mushrooms, oats, potatoes, avocados, brown rice, black beans

FAT-SOLUBLE VITAMINS

- **Vitamin A** Supports immune system function and vision. Contributes to cell renewal.
- **Vitamin D** A hormone produced in the kidneys by exposure to sunlight. Needed for the growth, development, and maintenance of strong teeth, bones, and muscles (see pp.104–105).
- **Vitamin E** A powerful antioxidant to protect cells from damage. It helps maintain healthy skin and eyes and strengthens the immune system.
- **Vitamin K** Needed to help blood clot.

MINERALS

- **Calcium** Keeps bones and teeth healthy. Important in muscle contraction, including the heart and for normal blood clotting (see pp.100–101).
- **Iodine** Needed for thyroid hormone production, brain development, and bone maintenance (see pp.108–109).
- **Iron** Needed to make red blood cells and help with immune and brain function (see pp.98–99).
- **Magnesium** Important for nervous system function and releasing energy from foods.
- **Phosphorous** Releases energy from food and builds and maintains strong teeth and bones.
- **Potassium** Regulates water content and maintains blood pressure. Helps functioning of the heart.
- **Selenium** Needed to protect cells from damage, supports immune function, supports normal fertility particularly in males (see pp.106–107).
- **Sodium** Regulates body water content.
- **Zinc** Supports immune system function, hormone and cell production, maintenance of skin, hair, and nails (see pp.112–113).

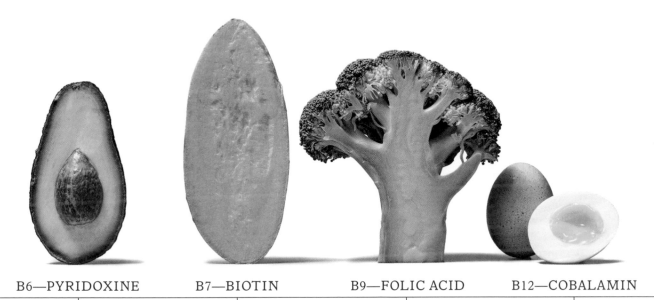

B6—PYRIDOXINE

Plant sources
Avocados, bananas, green vegetables, soy beans, quinoa, sunflower seeds

B7—BIOTIN

Plant sources
Found in most foods, including sweet potatoes

B9—FOLIC ACID

Plant sources
Broccoli, cabbage, kale, sprouts, chickpeas, kidney beans

B12—COBALAMIN

Animal and plant sources
Eggs, milk, fish, cheese, fortified yeast extract, cereals

WHAT ROLE DOES HYDRATION PLAY?

Water is essential for our survival and is often taken for granted, particularly in the Western world where we have easy access to plenty of clean drinking water. You need to drink enough water each day to stay alive and perform your daily tasks.

Every part of your body needs water to function, and it's vital to keep your fluid levels topped off. Water helps support essential systems, including the circulatory and digestive systems, and the brain.

WATER FROM FOOD

Up to 30 percent of our daily water intake can come from food, so it's important to include foods with a high water volume in your diet, especially when it's hot. There are a variety of foods that are hydrating. Many fruits and vegetables contain a lot of water, in particular strawberries, watermelon, peaches, cucumber, lettuce, tomatoes, and citrus fruits.

DRINKING FLUIDS

The other 70 percent of our daily water intake comes from drinking plenty of fluids throughout the day. In the US, the recommended amount is broken down into gender, with men being advised to

consume 125oz (3.7l) each day and women 91oz (2.7l). In the UK, 6–8 glasses a day (1.5–2l) is set as a target. Sadly, even with access to clean drinking water, 80 percent of people do not get enough, raising the risk of dehydration, fatigue, and heat stroke. The human body is 60 percent water, and we need to consistently ensure fluid levels remain optimal in order to feel well and stay healthy.

WHAT TO DRINK

● **Water** Tap water is safe in the US and in many other countries, but check the safety of supplies if you are traveling to new places.
● **Milk** Dairy or plant milks can be consumed as part of your daily intake.
● **Fruit juice** Limit to 4oz a day as it contains high levels of sugar.
● **Tea and coffee** Can contribute toward your daily hydration levels. Although both tea and coffee act as a diuretics (causing your body to excrete more water), this does not outweigh the hydration you can get from these drinks. You can include both the regular caffeinated or decaffeinated versions.
● **Unsweetened drinks** Unsweetened carbonated water counts.

TRY TO AVOID

● Sugar sweetened carbonated drinks.
● Too many drinks with artificial sweeteners—there is now emerging evidence these may not be good for our gut bugs.
● Too many caffeinated drinks (five or more cups of coffee a day, for example) can lead to dehydration.

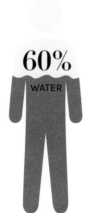

60% WATER

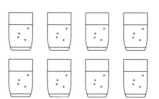

Keeping count One way to keep on top of hydration is to always keep a bottle of water with you at home or on the go and set yourself the target of drinking eight glasses of water a day.

DRINK 8+ GLASSES A DAY TO KEEP FLUID LEVELS OPTIMAL

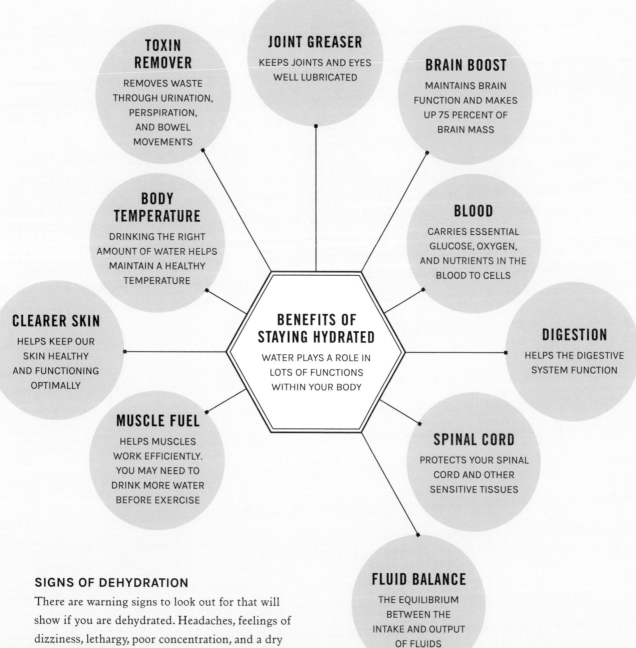

TOXIN REMOVER
REMOVES WASTE THROUGH URINATION, PERSPIRATION, AND BOWEL MOVEMENTS

JOINT GREASER
KEEPS JOINTS AND EYES WELL LUBRICATED

BRAIN BOOST
MAINTAINS BRAIN FUNCTION AND MAKES UP 75 PERCENT OF BRAIN MASS

BODY TEMPERATURE
DRINKING THE RIGHT AMOUNT OF WATER HELPS MAINTAIN A HEALTHY TEMPERATURE

BLOOD
CARRIES ESSENTIAL GLUCOSE, OXYGEN, AND NUTRIENTS IN THE BLOOD TO CELLS

CLEARER SKIN
HELPS KEEP OUR SKIN HEALTHY AND FUNCTIONING OPTIMALLY

BENEFITS OF STAYING HYDRATED
WATER PLAYS A ROLE IN LOTS OF FUNCTIONS WITHIN YOUR BODY

DIGESTION
HELPS THE DIGESTIVE SYSTEM FUNCTION

MUSCLE FUEL
HELPS MUSCLES WORK EFFICIENTLY. YOU MAY NEED TO DRINK MORE WATER BEFORE EXERCISE

SPINAL CORD
PROTECTS YOUR SPINAL CORD AND OTHER SENSITIVE TISSUES

FLUID BALANCE
THE EQUILIBRIUM BETWEEN THE INTAKE AND OUTPUT OF FLUIDS

SIGNS OF DEHYDRATION

There are warning signs to look out for that will show if you are dehydrated. Headaches, feelings of dizziness, lethargy, poor concentration, and a dry mouth are common symptoms. You may also notice that your urine is dark yellow. When you are well hydrated, your urine will be almost clear in color. Watch out for more serious chronic symptoms of dehydration like constipation, which can lead to urinary tract infections and the formation of kidney stones. Often, we don't realize we haven't had enough water before we notice any of these problems. Remember, when you exercise or you're in a hot climate where you sweat more, your requirements may also be higher.

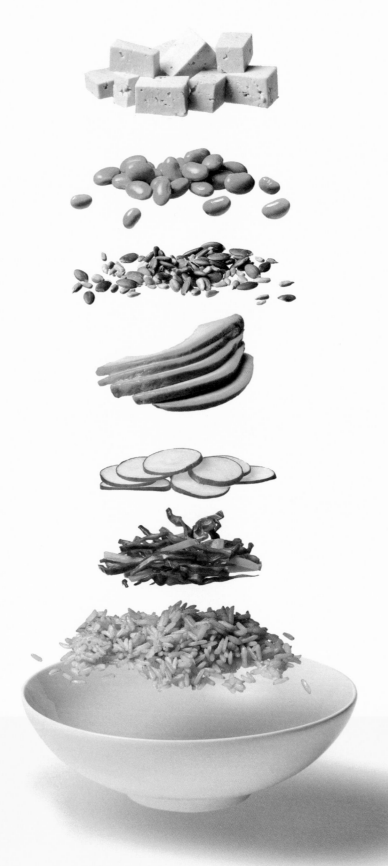

PROTEIN

PLANT SOURCES
INCLUDE TOFU, SEEDS,
AND EDAMAME BEANS.
THIS CAN MAKE UP
A QUARTER OF
THE MEAL.

FATS

INCLUDE HEALTHY FATS
FROM PLANT SOURCES
SUCH AS SEEDS.

VEGGIES & FRUITS

AROUND HALF OF ANY
MEAL SHOULD CONSIST
OF MICRONUTRIENT-
RICH FRESH FRUITS
AND VEGETABLES.

STARCHES

STARCHY CARBS ARE
A VITAL ENERGY SOURCE.
CHOOSE WHOLE
GRAIN RICE, BREAD,
AND PASTA.

The plant-based balanced plate
The "balanced plate" concept is a useful guide
to the types and proportions of foods we
should try to consume at mealtimes; apply it
when shopping, cooking, or eating out. It isn't
essential to achieve the balance of food groups
at every meal; just aim for it over the course of
your day or week.

WHAT ARE THE BASICS OF HEALTHY NUTRITION?

"Healthy" looks different to everyone. For some, it may be eating more greens; for others, it might be cooking from scratch for the first time. With so much information and conflicting theories, we can end up confused and frustrated. But the basic principles are very simple: variety and balance.

We must eat to survive, but for healthy dietary habits to become an integral part of our daily lives, food needs to be enjoyed. Satiation—comfortably satisfying feelings of hunger—is vitally important. The sociable aspects of eating are also important in creating long-term healthy behaviors. We can easily get caught up in the latest trends or number counting, but diet is so much more than numbers. Healthy doesn't have to be complicated—you won't find it in the latest diet book or trend; it's often going back to basics and educating yourself on the first principles of nutrition and applying it to your situation.

DAILY NEEDS

Food is fuel and satisfies the nutritional needs of a healthy body. A healthy adult's plant-based diet should contain a balance of carbohydrates, protein, and fat drawn from these key food groups: fresh fruit and vegetables; whole grain starchy carbohydrates like brown rice; mainly plant proteins such as tofu; healthy fats such as avocado and sources of omega-3 such as nuts and seeds. These macronutrients are required to provide energy and cellular building blocks for the functioning of the body's systems (see pp.20–21).

THE SPICE OF LIFE

Eating a variety of foods is one of the best ways to ensure you stay optimally healthy (see pp.66–73). No single food or food group can provide everything we need to remain fit and well, which is where variety comes in. Aim for a colorful array of fruits and vegetables daily, to ensure you obtain the widest range of micronutrients (vitamins and minerals). And these can be from frozen, fresh, or canned options—healthy eating doesn't have to be expensive.

WHOLE FOODS

Eating whole foods is a great way to enhance the fiber content in your diet and minimize a lot of extra and often unnecessary saturated fats, salt, sugar, and additives found in ultra-processed foods (see pp.30–31). The more you can cook a whole food diet from scratch, the better this will be for your health, as you'll know what is going into your body and be able to control any extras. Moderation is key, and allowing yourself "treat" items means you're less likely to overindulge. Any form of restriction is often mentally challenging for long-term healthy eating behaviors.

Where our food energy is needed

Food provides the body with fuel, and the major share of this energy is needed simply to keep the body ticking over and functioning properly.

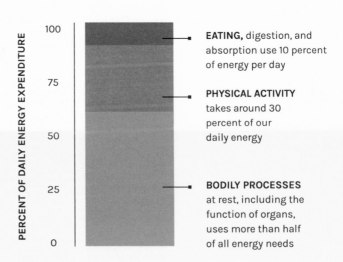

PERCENT OF DAILY ENERGY EXPENDITURE

100

75

50

25

0

EATING, digestion, and absorption use 10 percent of energy per day

PHYSICAL ACTIVITY takes around 30 percent of our daily energy

BODILY PROCESSES at rest, including the function of organs, uses more than half of all energy needs

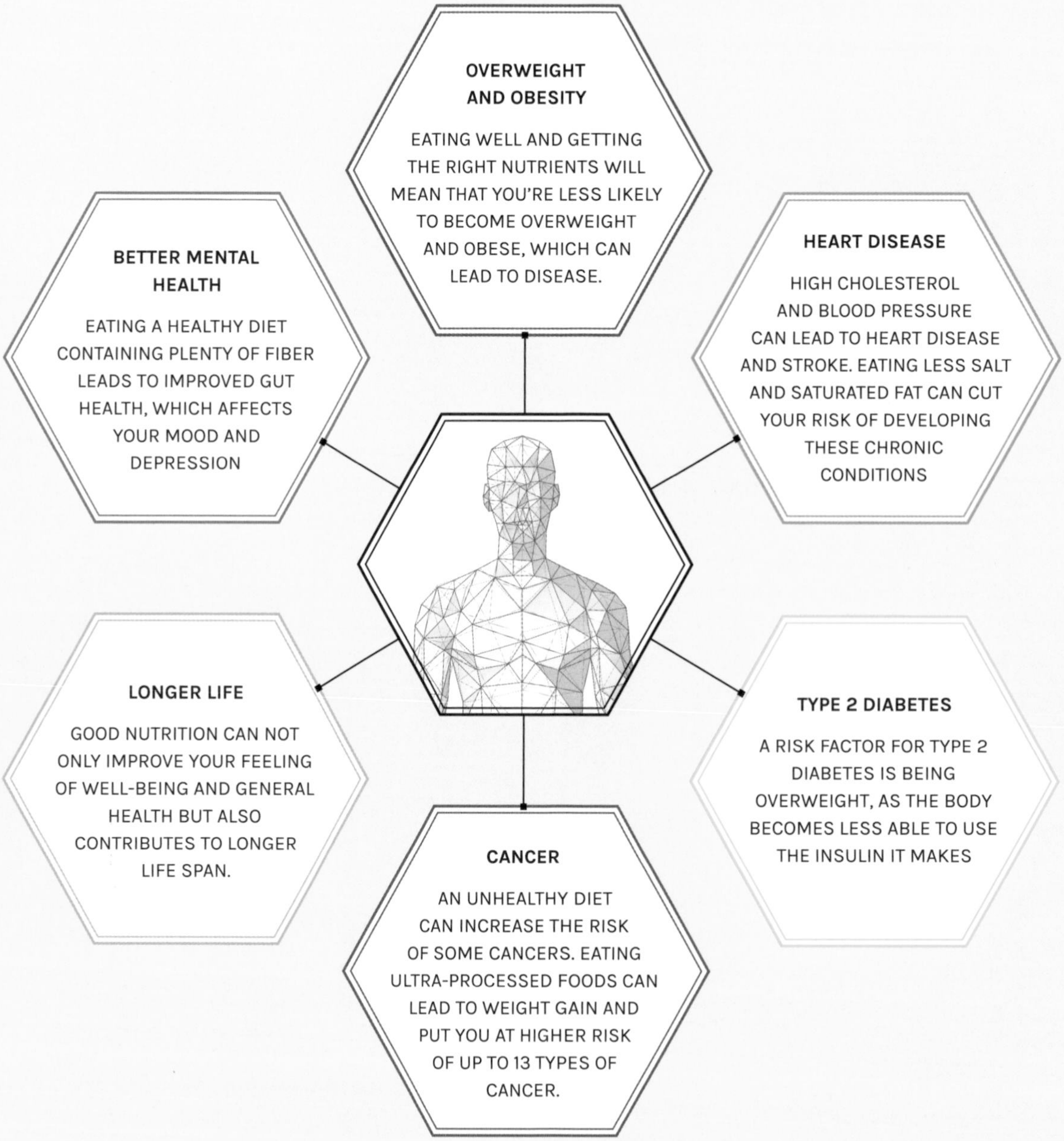

OVERWEIGHT AND OBESITY

EATING WELL AND GETTING THE RIGHT NUTRIENTS WILL MEAN THAT YOU'RE LESS LIKELY TO BECOME OVERWEIGHT AND OBESE, WHICH CAN LEAD TO DISEASE.

BETTER MENTAL HEALTH

EATING A HEALTHY DIET CONTAINING PLENTY OF FIBER LEADS TO IMPROVED GUT HEALTH, WHICH AFFECTS YOUR MOOD AND DEPRESSION

HEART DISEASE

HIGH CHOLESTEROL AND BLOOD PRESSURE CAN LEAD TO HEART DISEASE AND STROKE. EATING LESS SALT AND SATURATED FAT CAN CUT YOUR RISK OF DEVELOPING THESE CHRONIC CONDITIONS

LONGER LIFE

GOOD NUTRITION CAN NOT ONLY IMPROVE YOUR FEELING OF WELL-BEING AND GENERAL HEALTH BUT ALSO CONTRIBUTES TO LONGER LIFE SPAN.

CANCER

AN UNHEALTHY DIET CAN INCREASE THE RISK OF SOME CANCERS. EATING ULTRA-PROCESSED FOODS CAN LEAD TO WEIGHT GAIN AND PUT YOU AT HIGHER RISK OF UP TO 13 TYPES OF CANCER.

TYPE 2 DIABETES

A RISK FACTOR FOR TYPE 2 DIABETES IS BEING OVERWEIGHT, AS THE BODY BECOMES LESS ABLE TO USE THE INSULIN IT MAKES

Your overall health and life expectancy will be better if you consume a healthy, well-balanced diet containing plenty of fruits, vegetables, whole grains, beans, and pulses.

WHAT ARE THE BENEFITS OF GOOD NUTRITION?

Good nutrition positively affects how you perform and feel every day; it will also help keep you free from deficiencies, fight off illness, and reduce your risk of many ailments.

FEWER DISEASES

Healthy eating has a multitude of benefits for adults and children. The first being long life—better nutrition, research suggests, means that you are less likely to die from cancer, cardiovascular disease, and respiratory or neurodegenerative disease. Good nutrition will automatically lower your type 2 diabetes. This research is based on those who consume a diet containing plenty of whole grains, fruits, vegetables, nuts, and legumes. Another benefit of good nutrition is a healthy, optimally functioning digestive system, which, in turn, will help you maintain a healthy weight. Your gut health and immune system will be improved if you eat a diverse range of plants and a healthy diet (see pp.184–185).

While there are endless benefits to eating well, not all countries have access to good nutrition, leading to increased rates of infectious diseases and deficiencies, such as rickets. In western societies in recent years, we have seen a rise in people living with obesity, which increases their risk of disease (see pp.204–205).

TEETH, SKIN, AND MOUTH

An array of key vitamins, such as calcium, vitamin D, and phosphorus, and a diet that does not include too many food types and nutrients that contribute to tooth decay are needed to keep your teeth strong. There is also research that suggests that some cheese is beneficial for your teeth. Cheese is high in phosphate content, which helps balance pH levels in the mouth, and so can help preserve tooth enamel. The skin and mouth have their own microbiomes (see pp.206–207), which require a variety of vegetables, fruits, nuts, seeds, and pulses to stay healthy. Our skin and eyes require key nutrients found in a healthy diet rich in antioxidants, vitamins, minerals, and healthy fats.

MUSCLES AND BONES

A healthy diet can support your muscles. Skeletal muscle is highly sensitive to the nutrients we ea,t and your diet can impact the growth or maintenance of this tissue. Protein each day with the essential amino acids will help keep your muscles healthy, alongside lifestyle factors. Your bones require nutritional support to stay strong—vitamin K and calcium are both important for bone health (see pp.186–187).

Mental health

WHILE THERE ARE MANY MEASURABLE BENEFITS TO EATING A GOOD DIET, OTHERS ARE MORE DIFFICULT TO QUANTIFY, SUCH AS MOOD.
When you don't eat enough nutrient-rich foods, your body may lack vital vitamins and minerals, which may affect your energy, mood, and brain function. Eating regularly throughout the day helps maintain stable blood sugar levels, which also affects your concentration and the way you feel (see pp.172-173). Furthermore, research has now confirmed that the gut-brain axis plays a role in mental health. The first study in the world to demonstrate that making dietary changes can be effective in improving mental health is called the SMILES trial (see pp.178-179).

HOW CAN I AVOID POOR NUTRITION?

Poor nutrition can also be referred to as malnutrition, which can be serious and in some cases life threatening. It is usually caused by not eating enough of the right foods to keep your body healthy. Malnutrition can also be caused by overeating, which can lead to obesity.

To be healthy and eat well, you need to strike a balance between the types of foods you consume commonly for enjoyment compared to those that are necessary. Food should be enjoyed, but there is a rising rate of obesity as a result of poor nutrition.

UNDERNUTRITION

Poor nutrition can be caused by many different factors. Undernutrition is caused by not consuming enough nutrients and can result in losing weight and being underweight. It can also occur when we don't get the right micronutrients (see pp.22–23). The most common nutrient deficiencies worldwide are in iron, vitamin A, and iodine. Most of these problems occur in low- and middle-income populations and they have long-term impacts for the individuals as well as for the country as a whole. Around 45 percent of child deaths worldwide under the age of five are caused by undernutrition. At the same time, the numbers of children who are overweight and obese are rising as ultra-processed foods become more available and are consumed as the main source of nutrition. If you consume too much energy for your body over a period of time, it can lead to weight gain and poor nutrient absorption (see pp.204–205). Malnutrition can be caused by too little or too much food and causes many health issues. Globally in 2020, 149 million children under five were estimated to be stunted (too short for age), 45 million were estimated to be wasted (too thin for height), and 38.9 million were overweight or obese.

ULTRA-PROCESSED FOOD

Higher rates of obesity are being fueled by an increase in ultra-processed food, also referred to as convenience food, fast food, or junk food. Foods like this are often more energy-dense than unprocessed foods and contains high levels of sugar and fat. It's also worth remembering that some plant-based foods are ultra-processed (see pp.60–61).

What you can do

If you are fortunate enough to have access to good food and nutritional education, keep an eye on your intake of salt, fat, and sugar and avoid ultra-processed foods where possible.

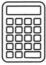

CALORIES

Ensure your food is not too high or too low in calories to meet your energy requirements. Calories are rough measures of energy but can be helpful in this instance.

SALT

Check that you are not eating more than the recommended <2,300mg of salt a day within your diet.

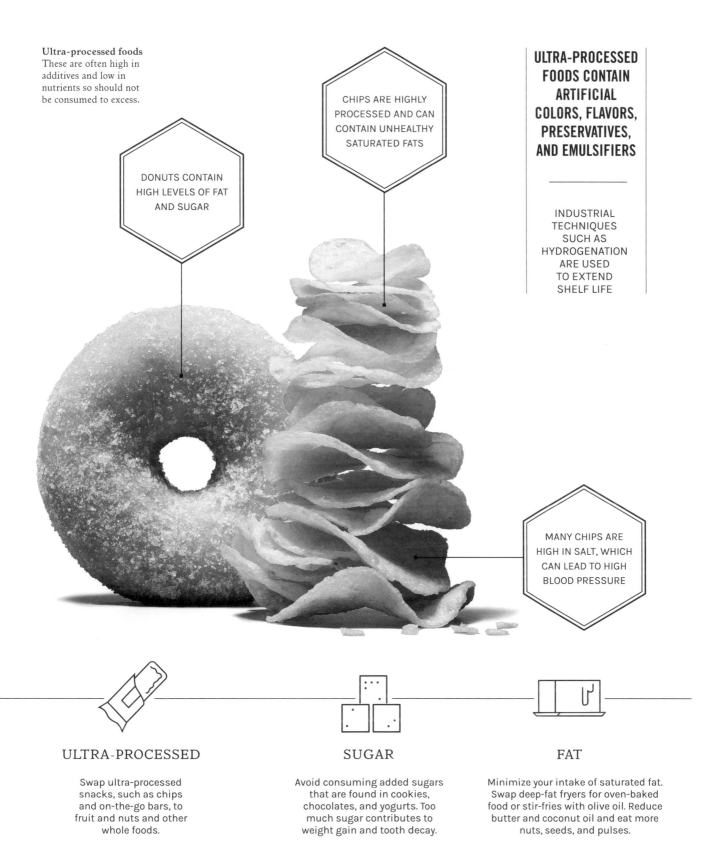

Ultra-processed foods
These are often high in additives and low in nutrients so should not be consumed to excess.

CHIPS ARE HIGHLY PROCESSED AND CAN CONTAIN UNHEALTHY SATURATED FATS

ULTRA-PROCESSED FOODS CONTAIN ARTIFICIAL COLORS, FLAVORS, PRESERVATIVES, AND EMULSIFIERS

INDUSTRIAL TECHNIQUES SUCH AS HYDROGENATION ARE USED TO EXTEND SHELF LIFE

DONUTS CONTAIN HIGH LEVELS OF FAT AND SUGAR

MANY CHIPS ARE HIGH IN SALT, WHICH CAN LEAD TO HIGH BLOOD PRESSURE

ULTRA-PROCESSED

Swap ultra-processed snacks, such as chips and on-the-go bars, to fruit and nuts and other whole foods.

SUGAR

Avoid consuming added sugars that are found in cookies, chocolates, and yogurts. Too much sugar contributes to weight gain and tooth decay.

FAT

Minimize your intake of saturated fat. Swap deep-fat fryers for oven-baked food or stir-fries with olive oil. Reduce butter and coconut oil and eat more nuts, seeds, and pulses.

HOW DOES POOR NUTRITION IMPACT HEALTH?

The diet you consume has the potential to impact your health.
In fact, a childhood diet lacking the necessary vitamins and minerals, despite adequate calories, can cause irreversible damage that has educational, financial, and long-term health consequences reaching far into adulthood.

Many conditions are closely linked with the diets we consume, and research is now suggesting lifestyle factors can play a role in preventing disease and illness. Diet can help decrease the risk of poor health, from cancers to heart disease, and the correct nutrition can shape positive mental health outcomes.

DIABETES

More than 500,000 participants from six different countries took part in a study looking at the risk of type 2 diabetes. An increased risk was shown with the consumption of sugar-sweetened beverages, red meat, processed meat, and lack of fiber while a decreased risk occurred when consuming whole grains, fruits, and dairy. Today's diet high in ultra-processed foods alongside things like age, ethnicity, and family history can all contribute to overall risk. Obesity is one of the most significant risk factors, although not everyone who is at risk or living with type 2 diabetes is carrying extra weight.

CANCERS

Consuming unhealthy sugar-sweetened drinks and highly processed food can lead to weight gain, obesity, and other chronic conditions that put people at higher risk of at least 13 types of cancer. These include endometrial (uterine) cancer, breast cancer in postmenopausal women, and colorectal cancer. Eating a healthy diet helps you maintain a healthy weight, or lose weight, which can reduce the risk of developing these diseases. Although we know that some key food items—processed and red meat,

alcohol, high calorie foods, and sugary drinks—are directly linked to an increased risk of cancer, it is thought that your overall diet has a bigger impact on cancer risk than individual foods. Eating a small amount of processed and red meat, therefore, is less harmful than eating a poor diet lacking in plants and whole foods over a period of time.

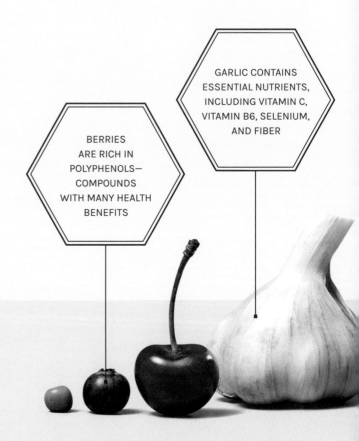

GARLIC CONTAINS ESSENTIAL NUTRIENTS, INCLUDING VITAMIN C, VITAMIN B6, SELENIUM, AND FIBER

BERRIES ARE RICH IN POLYPHENOLS— COMPOUNDS WITH MANY HEALTH BENEFITS

HEART HEALTH

Poor diets high in saturated fat, salt, and too many calories are linked to heart disease (see pp.190–191). Trials including participants who were either healthy or had higher cholesterol levels found that substituting plant-based proteins like beans and lentils for red meat reduced risk factors for heart disease. Poor diets high in ultra-processed foods (see pp. 30–31) often have high levels of saturated fat. This can increase the amount of cholesterol in the blood, increasing the risk of coronary heart disease.

IMMUNITY

A poor diet lacking key nutrients can contribute to a weakened immune system. Inflammation (a type of immune response) can be influenced by diet, and studies have reported that diets high in fruits and vegetables, whole grains, and healthy fats, and low in refined carbs, fried foods, sugar-sweetened beverages, and red and processed meats may help reduce the risk of inflammation. Seventy percent of our immune system resides in our gut so by improving our diets and gut health, we can help our immune system (see pp.184–185).

Depression and anxiety

PROBLEMS LIKE DEPRESSION AND ANXIETY MAY BE ASSOCIATED WITH POOR DIETS.
There is evidence to suggest that pathways related to cell damage, inflammation, cell energy dysfunction, and gut microbiota disorders are disrupted in those with mental health disorders. Dietary interventions may improve mental well-being by reducing the consumption of foods associated with increased risk for depression, such as processed meats and refined carbohydrates.

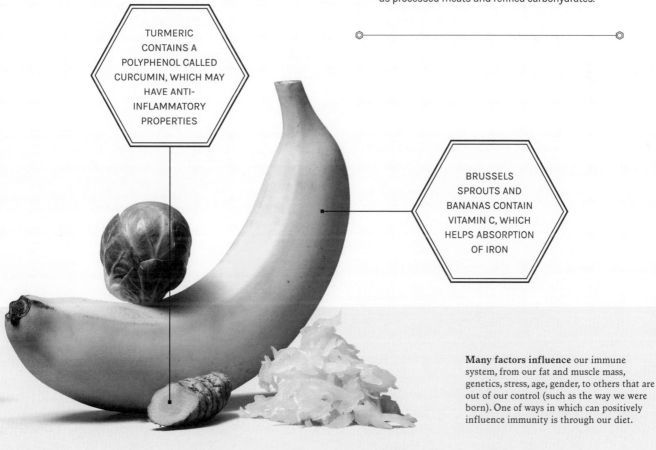

TURMERIC CONTAINS A POLYPHENOL CALLED CURCUMIN, WHICH MAY HAVE ANTI-INFLAMMATORY PROPERTIES

BRUSSELS SPROUTS AND BANANAS CONTAIN VITAMIN C, WHICH HELPS ABSORPTION OF IRON

Many factors influence our immune system, from our fat and muscle mass, genetics, stress, age, gender, to others that are out of our control (such as the way we were born). One of ways in which can positively influence immunity is through our diet.

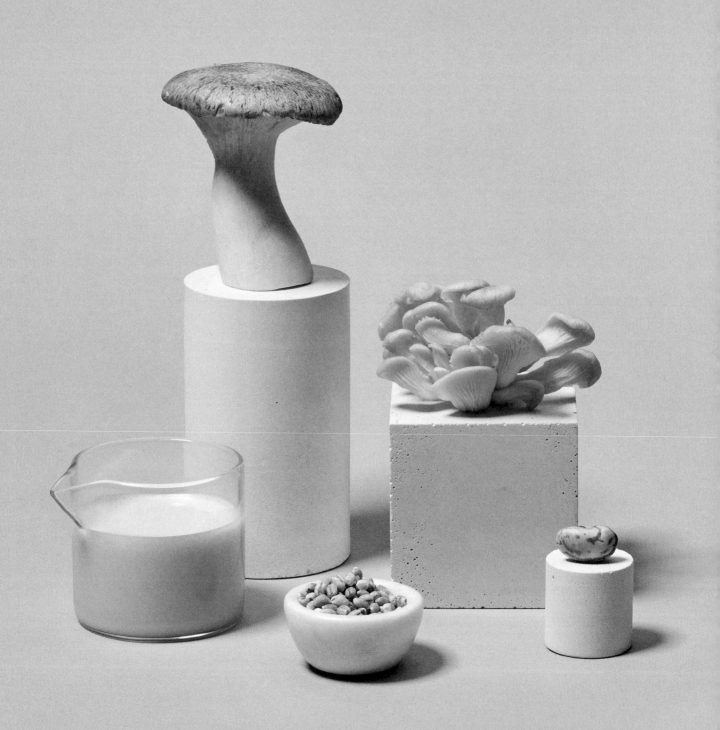

INTRODUCING PLANT-BASED NUTRITION

WHAT DOES PLANT-BASED ACTUALLY MEAN?

"Plant-based" has entered common parlance in recent years, but people often use it interchangeably with veganism, when, in fact, the term encompasses a much broader range of dietary choices.

To put it simply, plant-based eating means incorporating predominantly plants into your diet, not only fruits and vegetables but also nuts, seeds, whole grains, legumes, and beans. At its simplest, enjoying a plant-based diet means eating more plants and fewer animal products, with the aim of obtaining the majority of your nutritional needs from plants and whole foods. Unlike plant-based eating, veganism is the complete omission from the diet of animal produce and anything derived from animals. Vegans also sometimes make wider consumer choices, such as avoiding leather products.

	PLANTS	EGGS	DAIRY	FISH	MEAT
VEGAN					
LACTO VEGAN					
OVO VEGETARIAN					
VEGETARIAN					
PESCATARIAN					
FLEXITARIAN					
OMNIVORE					

EMBRACING WHOLE FOOD DIVERSITY

Another way of approaching plant-based eating is as a way to aim for a whole food diet that embraces color, variety, taste, and texture and with this a new food repertoire, moving away from ultra-processed convenience options and creating more meals from scratch at home where possible. Although there are now more ready-made plant-based options available to buy in our supermarkets than ever before, these are not always the healthiest option (see pp.60–61).

IMPACT ON HEALTH

If followed correctly, plant-based eating may have a positive impact on your health and potentially the planet (see pp.42–45). The research supporting the beneficial outcomes of eating in this way is growing, with evidence that it can help lower greenhouse gas emissions and have positive outcomes on our health, such as reducing our risk of heart disease and type 2 diabetes. As with every area of science, particularly in nutrition, there are different schools of thought. Some scientists believe that one way of eating is the gold standard for us all. This is, of course, incorrect; there is no one size that fits all when it comes to diet, but making informed choices and choosing a diet that works for you is often the best approach.

PLANT-BASED DIET DIVERSITY

From omnivore to vegan and everything in between, anyone can be a plant-based eater. The unifying factor is that you are satisfying the overwhelming majority of your nutritional needs by eating the widest variety of plants and plant-derived foods.

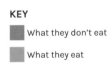

KEY

What they don't eat

What they eat

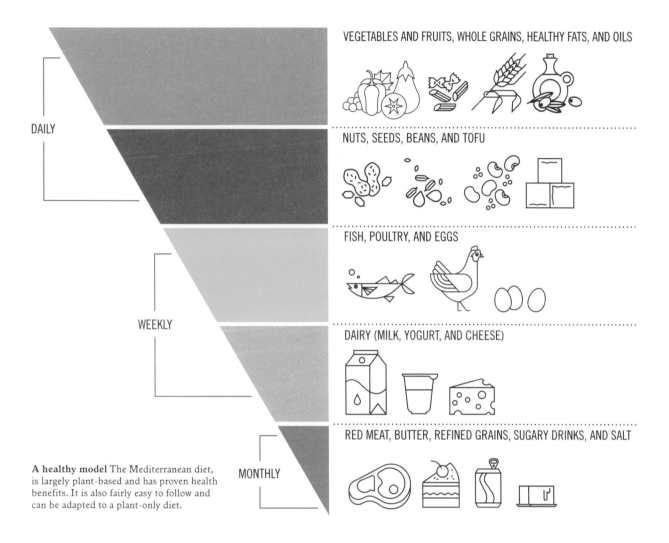

DAILY

VEGETABLES AND FRUITS, WHOLE GRAINS, HEALTHY FATS, AND OILS

NUTS, SEEDS, BEANS, AND TOFU

WEEKLY

FISH, POULTRY, AND EGGS

DAIRY (MILK, YOGURT, AND CHEESE)

RED MEAT, BUTTER, REFINED GRAINS, SUGARY DRINKS, AND SALT

MONTHLY

A healthy model The Mediterranean diet, is largely plant-based and has proven health benefits. It is also fairly easy to follow and can be adapted to a plant-only diet.

The Mediterranean diet

IN MANY WAYS, OUR UNDERSTANDING OF THE BENEFITS OF PLANT-BASED EATING IS NOTHING NEW.

The idea of the Mediterranean diet as a model of healthy nutrition dates from the 1960s, and it is largely plant-based. This way of eating is low in saturated fat and high in vegetable oils and is traditionally common in olive-growing countries within the Mediterranean region. While the diet has many definitions, they are all based around the same components: a high intake of plant foods, such as whole grains, fruits, vegetables, nuts, pulses, legumes, and extra-virgin olive oil; moderate intakes of dairy products, poultry, fish, and occasional good quality red wine; and low intakes of saturated fats, red meat, and sugary foods. Much of the research highlights the many benefits of eating this way, including lower rates of cardiovascular disease, diabetes, obesity, certain cancers, and better cognitive and mental function.

WHY ARE PEOPLE GOING VEGAN?

During the time that humans have been on Earth, we have mainly eaten a plant-based diet due to the fact that it is easier to get hold of fresh fruit, nuts, leaves, and seeds than to catch and eat meat. More meat has been consumed over the last 50 years as it has become cheaper, but increasing numbers of people are now turning to veganism.

Vegans don't eat anything that comes from animals, including eggs, milk, and honey. Many also choose not to buy clothes or shoes made from leather or to use any products such as toiletries that are made using animal products. Plant-based eaters, on the other hand, mainly eat fruits, vegetables, whole grains, beans, nuts, and seeds but may still consume some animal products (see pp.36–37). Currently, it is believed that 1 in 10 Americans consider themselves vegan, while the numbers in Europe are also on the rise. The rise of flexitarian diets could well be here to stay, with 55 percent of Germans having reduced meat intake and in the UK 46 percent of British adults considering reducing their intake of animal products in the future. There are several reasons why people choose to go vegan.

ETHICAL REASONS

Many choose to eat a vegan diet in order to spare the suffering caused to animals in the modern food production process. Although we may like to think that animals are able to enjoy a long and happy life before dying in a humane fashion, sadly this is often not the case. Some animals, such as chickens, are bred to gain weight quickly so they reach the right size for the food industry. Many spend shortened lives in overcrowded and unnatural conditions before heading for the slaughterhouse.

HEALTH BENEFITS

Avoiding overconsumption of meat and dairy is known to have many long-term health benefits, although it is important to remember that not all vegans are healthy. It is perfectly possible to be a vegan who eats overprocessed foods containing too much salt, sugar, and fat. However, there is research to show that vegans may have a reduced risk of heart disease and type 2 diabetes as well as protection from some cancers, in particular, colorectal cancer, which is linked with overconsumption of red meat.

ENVIRONMENTAL REASONS

Many people are now choosing to go vegan to help limit the damage our actions are having on wildlife and the natural world. Eating meat has a huge effect on the planet, with some estimating that the production of animal food is responsible for 14.5 percent of planet-heating gases caused by humans. Beef production is the worst offender out of all food products, with lamb and dairy just behind. Some of the pollution is caused by the emissions from the animals themselves, but other factors include deforestation (to make way for farmland) and flying and shipping refrigerated foods around the world. Harm is also caused by the amount of food that is wasted in our current systems. Farm waste in particular affects the oceans, damaging fish, and causing the extinction of many sea creatures.

University of Oxford research concluded that adopting a plant-based diet can reduce our own food emissions by 73 percent, depending on where we live. A plant-based diet isn't the same as a vegan diet as it can contain some meat and dairy products, while being mainly based on plant foods.

DAIRY
Contributes to 14.3% of greenhouse gas emissions of total dietary intake.

DEPLETED FISH STOCKS
90%
of fisheries are now fully exploited

FINANCIAL
Eating a vegan diet can be cheaper than a meat or fish diet.

ANIMAL WELFARE
A major concern for many people is the way that animals in the food chain are treated.

GREENHOUSE GAS EMISSIONS
Cattle are responsible for
62%
of food emissions

EFFECTS OF OVERFISHING
Fishing has caused damage to the marine ecosystem.

WHY EAT VEGAN?
THERE ARE MANY REASONS WHY PEOPLE CHOOSE TO GO VEGAN

HEALTH
A vegan diet is generally low in saturated fat and cholesterol and high in fiber.

WATER USE
Our current food systems account for 70% of all human water use.

CARBON FOOTPRINT
Reducing consumption of meat and dairy products would help reduce emissions.

WATER POLLUTION
Manure from cattle is a source of pollution to waterways.

ENVIRONMENT
Beef consumption contributes 16.2% of dietary greenhouse gas emissions, lamb 3.8%, and white meat 4.1%.

BIODIVERSITY
In the US, industrialized livestock production is directly responsible for 85% of all soil erosion..

The vegan choice Increasing numbers of people globally are adopting veganism for a wide variety of reasons.

HOW CAN I TELL WHAT IS AND ISN'T PLANT-BASED?

You may be completely vegan or you may be eating a plant-based diet, but it's not always easy to know whether the food you're buying contains any animal products. Checking the label is the easiest way to know, but there are other things to look out for.

CHECK THE LABEL

It is up to you how far you decide to stick to the vegan or plant-based lifestyle, you may be relaxed about certain animal products or you may decide that you will avoid animal products altogether. Particularly if you're on the go, it can be difficult to know all the ingredients of a food product. So much of what we eat contains animal products, even if it's not immediately obvious. The only way to be sure of the ingredients of any food is to check the label.

Many companies in the US and in other countries have adopted vegan certification on packaging so you need to look out for a label that says "Suitable for vegans" or has a "Certified Vegan" logo. Another simple way is to scan the "Allergen Information." If the product contains dairy, eggs, or seafood, it will be stated under its allergen ingredients list. Different countries have different guidelines, but generally speaking, reading the labels is the only way to be truly sure that what you are eating is plant-based.

HIDDEN INGREDIENTS

It is worth knowing a little bit about the additives and hidden extras that are in so many of our everyday foods. Some everyday food that you may not think of as being nonvegan can have hidden animal-derived ingredients. One example of this is pesto, which contains Parmesan cheese, while some bakery products, such as bagels and breads, often contain added L-cysteine. This amino acid is used as a softening agent and often comes from poultry feathers or animal hair.

ADDITIVES DERIVED FROM ANIMALS

In the US and other countries, there are different systems for labeling additives, usually including the full name of the additive or product on the food label. In Europe, food additives must be marked on the ingredients list on food products and are given an E number. Some of the most commonly used additives that contain animal products are shown opposite. You may choose to avoid these if you're eating a plant-based diet.

Check the label

IF ANIMAL-DERIVED GELATIN IS INCLUDED IN ANY FOOD IT IS LISTED ON THE INGREDIENTS LABEL. Products can be tested for gelatin using DNA and antibody tests. The processing of the gelatin can make it difficult to detect as the DNA and protein structures are destroyed. New tests are being developed to overcome this problem.

INGREDIENTS: GLUCOSE SYRUP, SUGAR, GELATIN, DEXTROSE, CITRIC ACID, ARTIFICIAL AND NATURAL FLAVORS, PALM OIL, PALM KERNEL OIL, CARNAUBA WAX, WHITE BEESWAX, YELLOW BEESWAX, YELLOW 5, RED 40, BLUE 1

Gummy candies typically contain gelatin

Animal-based products commonly found in food and beauty products

There are many products to look out for if you are avoiding all animal products in food. Some of these you may recognize, while others are not so well known. There are too many items to list in this book, which emphasizes the degree to which we rely upon animal produce, from the food we eat to the clothes we wear.

Gelatin is a thickening agent used in jello. It comes from the skin, bones, and connective tissues of cows and pigs.

Cochineal or carmine is a natural dye made from insects, used to give a red color to many foods.

Lactitol is a sweetener derived from lactose (made from milk). Used in ice creams, sweets, and baked goods.

Beeswax is a wax made by bees and used as a glazing agent. Sometimes used to coat breads and pastries.

L-cysteine made from animal hair and feathers. Used in some breads as a proving agent.

Bone phosphate comes from the bones of cattle or pigs. Used in some dry foods to prevent them from sticking together.

Lanolin is a greasy substance secreted by sheep. It is used in some breastfeeding products.

Shellac A substance secreted by the female lac insect. Used to make a glaze or wax coating for food.

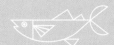

Cod liver oil is commonly used in omega-3 supplements, opt for algae instead (see pp.102–103).

Collagen is made from the skin, bones, and connective tissues of animals such as cows, chickens, pigs, and fish.

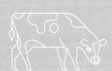

Elastin comes from cows' neck ligaments and aorta of. It is used in some cosmetics and skincare products.

Keratin is derived from the skin, bones, and connective tissues of animals and is used in some shampoos.

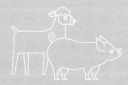

Lard and tallow is fatty tissue from animals. Lard is pork fat, while tallow is fat from cattle or sheep.

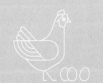

Albumen and albumin come from chickens. Albumen is egg white. Albumin is a protein made by the liver.

Isinglass is a gelatin-like substance derived from fish bladders. Often used to make beer or wine.

IS PLANT-BASED BETTER FOR A SUSTAINABLE FUTURE?

It may be better for our health to eat a plant-based diet, but is it better for the future of our planet? With around 30 percent of global greenhouse gas emissions coming from global food systems, changing our diet could make a significant difference. The challenge is to feed growing populations in a sustainable way.

WHAT IS A SUSTAINABLE DIET?

Sustainable diets are dietary patterns that promote all dimensions of an individual's health. The UN suggests a sustainable diet must support well-being, with a low environmental impact and pressure on the planet's resources that is cost effective and culturally acceptable. The global food system accounts for a third of emissions—this includes food production, processing, packaging, distribution, and consumption. It's also responsible for around 30 percent of global energy consumption. By 2030, it is estimated that 75 percent of warming caused by food production will be attributed to the production of high methane foods, such as meat, dairy, and rice.

All other food categories (such as vegetables, fruits, oils, grains, and seafood) contribute less than 5 percent each. Our global food system is also responsible for habitat loss, soil degradation, water usage, and waste (see pp.38–39).

CUTTING GREENHOUSE GASES

One study suggested that greenhouse gas emissions could be reduced by 22 percent by people moving to Mediterranean-style, pescatarian, vegetarian, and vegan diets. However, it is important to remember that not all plant food appears to be made equal when it comes to sustainable diets, rice being an important example. Rice production is currently responsible for 10 percent of global methane emissions, although initiatives are being developed to improve this. With less meat, would we rely even more on rice as a source of energy and protein?

CHANGING OUR HABITS

In order to reduce the emissions caused by food production, it will be necessary to change our diets and the way we see food. Recent research suggests that in order to reduce emissions, we need to double

PERCENTAGE OF GREENHOUSE GAS EMISSIONS (CO$_2$ eq) OF TOTAL DIETARY INTAKE

The production of red meat and diary products causes the most greenhouse emissions out of all food types.

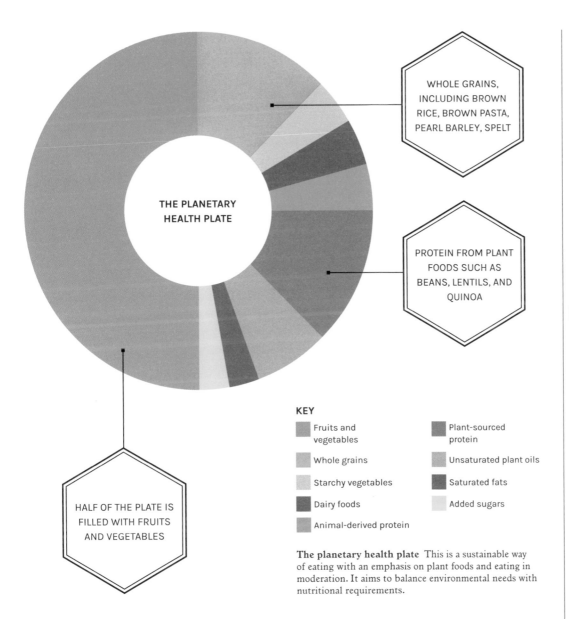

THE PLANETARY
HEALTH PLATE

WHOLE GRAINS,
INCLUDING BROWN
RICE, BROWN PASTA,
PEARL BARLEY, SPELT

PROTEIN FROM PLANT
FOODS SUCH AS
BEANS, LENTILS, AND
QUINOA

HALF OF THE PLATE IS
FILLED WITH FRUITS
AND VEGETABLES

KEY

- Fruits and vegetables
- Whole grains
- Starchy vegetables
- Dairy foods
- Animal-derived protein
- Plant-sourced protein
- Unsaturated plant oils
- Saturated fats
- Added sugars

The planetary health plate This is a sustainable way
of eating with an emphasis on plant foods and eating in
moderation. It aims to balance environmental needs with
nutritional requirements.

THE CLIMATE
CHANGE
COMMITTEE
RECOMMEND A
20%
SHIFT FROM MEAT
BY 2030

A 35%
REDUCTION
IN MEAT
CONSUMPTION
BY 2050 IS
RECOMMENDED

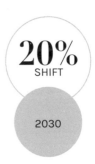

20%
SHIFT

2030

A 20% SHIFT FROM
DAIRY PRODUCTS
BY 2030 IS
RECOMMENDED
FOR A MORE
SUSTAINABLE
FOOD FUTURE

**A CUT IN MEAT
AND DAIRY
CONSUMPTION
COULD LEAD TO A
PER PERSON FALL
OF 5.5 TONS OF
CO$_2$ EMISSIONS**

our consumption of healthy plant-based foods,
such as fruits, vegetables, legumes, and nuts, and
cut by half our consumption of added sugars
and red meat.

At the same time, we need to ensure our diets
contain enough energy (calories) to sustain life.
Achieving a sustainable food system that can
deliver healthy diets for a growing world
population presents formidable challenges.
The planetary health plate is a way of

visualizing how a shift in our habits could look.
Although it still contains some dairy and meat
foods, half of the plate is given to fruits and
vegetables and most of the protein comes from
plant foods. These could be meat substitutes
such as tofu as well as plant foods like beans
and lentils. Whole grains make up another
substantial portion on the plate. Bear this in
mind when planning your meals, and you'll soon
be eating a more sustainable diet.

WHAT ARE THE NUTRITIONAL BENEFITS OF PLANT-BASED?

Plant-based diets can have a myriad of health benefits if followed sensibly. The main advantages of including more plants in your diet come with the increased fiber content and the reduction in saturated fat, but there are many other positives.

All the evidence we have points to the fact that eating plant-based can have a good effect on all areas of health. A 2019 study from the Journal of the American Heart Association found that middle-aged adults who ate diets high in healthful plant foods and low in animal products had a lower risk of heart disease. The American Heart Association states that eating less meat is associated with a lower risk of stroke, type 2 diabetes, high blood pressure, high cholesterol, some cancers, and obesity.

HEART HEALTH

Meat contains a lot of cholesterol and saturated fat, both of which are associated with heart disease. Processed meats like deli meat (for example, salami), ham, bacon, and sausages also contain high levels of salt, which can lead to high blood pressure. If you are keeping some meat in your diet, go for lean meats, skinless poultry, and fish as these can be good sources of protein in the correct amounts.

IMPROVING DIABETES

Researchers have looked at whether following a plant-based diet can help treat diabetes. A 2018 review suggested that vegetarian and vegan diets may be positive for people living with type 2 diabetes and reduce their medication needs, help them lose weight, and improve other metabolic markers. While veganism showed the most benefits, the researchers stated that all plant-based diets would lead to improvements by improving insulin sensitivity and reducing insulin resistance, but we need larger studies and more evidence in this area.

LOWER RATES OF OBESITY

A 2018 study found that a plant-based diet was effective for treating obesity (see pp.204–205). In the study, researchers assigned 75 people who were overweight or obese to follow either a vegan diet or to continue eating their regular diet, which contained meat. After four months, only the vegan group showed a significant weight loss of 14.33 pounds (6.5 kilograms). The plant-based vegan group also lost more fat mass and saw improvements in insulin sensitivity, whereas those who consumed a regular diet with meat did not. We have to remember, though, that you can be healthy with any dietary choice from plant-based to a diet containing meat. It all depends on the quantity and quality of the diet and other lifestyle factors such as exercise and sleep.

Dietary deficiencies

WHILE THERE ARE MANY HEALTHY BENEFITS ASSOCIATED WITH EATING A PLANT-BASED DIET, YOU SHOULD BE AWARE OF DIETARY CHOICES

It is possible to eat an unhealthy plant-based diet containing ultra-processed foods. It's important to eat a well-balanced and diverse diet that includes a variety of food types to make sure that you're meeting your nutritional needs. Certain needs cannot be met by eating plants alone so you may need to consider supplementation (see pp.96–97) and, in particular, vitamin B12, iodine, iron, calcium, and omega-3.

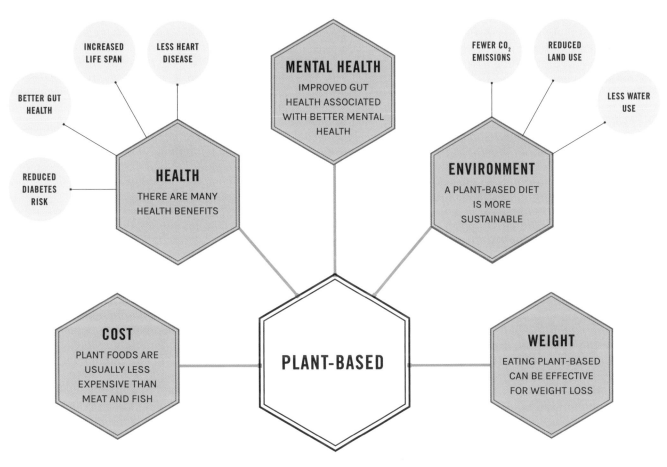

BETTER GUT HEALTH

INCREASED LIFE SPAN

LESS HEART DISEASE

REDUCED DIABETES RISK

HEALTH
THERE ARE MANY HEALTH BENEFITS

MENTAL HEALTH
IMPROVED GUT HEALTH ASSOCIATED WITH BETTER MENTAL HEALTH

FEWER CO$_2$ EMISSIONS

REDUCED LAND USE

LESS WATER USE

ENVIRONMENT
A PLANT-BASED DIET IS MORE SUSTAINABLE

COST
PLANT FOODS ARE USUALLY LESS EXPENSIVE THAN MEAT AND FISH

PLANT-BASED

WEIGHT
EATING PLANT-BASED CAN BE EFFECTIVE FOR WEIGHT LOSS

Advantages of eating a plant-based diet

There are many nutritional benefits of a plant-based diet. Knowing that you're helping the environment is also valuable.

GUT HEALTH STATS

One of the most important benefits of eating a plant-based diet is that it includes a higher intake of fiber, which supports a healthy gut microbiome. The American Gut Study, the largest published study to date of the human microbiome, found that people regularly eating more than 30 different types of plant foods each week (see pp.70–71) had a more diverse microbiome (see pp.22–23) than those eating 10 or fewer different plant foods a week. A diverse microbiome leads to better health outcomes because

of its positive effect on digestion, metabolism, and immune function. The compounds in plant foods (polyphenols and phytochemicals) may also improve the composition and activity of the gut microbiome.

INCREASED LIFE SPAN?

Research shows that reducing meat consumption may increase your life span by 3.6 years. It has also been found that societies with plant-based diets are more likely to live past 70 years, although other variables, such as healthcare, are also important.

ARE THERE ANY CONS TO A PLANT-BASED DIET?

There are many positive benefits from eating a plant-based diet, including to your health and for the environment. But are there any downsides to be aware of? Understanding the contribution that animal products make to the diet is an important part of understanding how to successfully eat a plant-based diet.

As with every dietary choice, it is important to be knowledgeable about what you are eating. Eating in a way that keeps you healthy is crucial, so you need to be aware of your nutritional needs. There are some key nutrients that may be lacking if you decide not to consume animal produce. You might need to add these by taking supplements (see pp. 96–97).

IRON INTAKE

If you cut meat from your diet, you need to consider your iron intake since red meat contains a high concentration of iron. One of the most common deficiencies is iron deficiency, and it is more common in lower income regions of sub-Saharan Africa, South Asia, and the Caribbean. It affects 2–5

percent of adult men and postmenopausal women and a higher number of women during childbearing years. The prevalence of iron-deficiency anemia is estimated to be 15 to 25 percent in pregnant women. This condition also affects 24 percent of the world's population, according to the World Health Organization. If you are eating a plant-based diet, you may need to take an iron supplement (see pp.98–99).

VITAMINS AND NUTRIENTS

Vitamins B12 and D are not found naturally in plant foods at all, and even if they are added to some fortified options, such as cereals, spreads, and meat alternatives, it is unlikely that you will get enough of them from diet alone (see pp.104–105 and 110–111). Dairy foods, such as milk and cheese, are perhaps one of the biggest contributors to many people's calcium intakes, particularly those of young children, so it's important to get that nutrient from other sources (see pp.100–101). Other nutrients that may be lacking are zinc (see pp.112–113), selenium (see pp.106–107), iodine (see pp.108–109), and omega-3 (see pp.102–103).

ARE MEAT ALTERNATIVES GOOD FOR YOU?

There is also an argument that eating more plant-based alternatives to meat options is not healthier as these "meat replacements" are often higher in added sugars and salt. Nearly three-quarters of plant-based meat alternatives exceed salt recommendations. Some studies have suggested that supplementing

ANEMIA AFFECTS AN ESTIMATED

1,620,000,000

PEOPLE OR ROUGHLY 24%

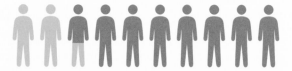

OF THE GLOBAL POPULATION

IRON DEFICIENCY
Lack of iron, often caused by inadequate dietary intake, is a common problem. If you eat a plant-based diet, you need to make sure to eat iron-rich foods such as lentils, spinach, tofu, and beans.

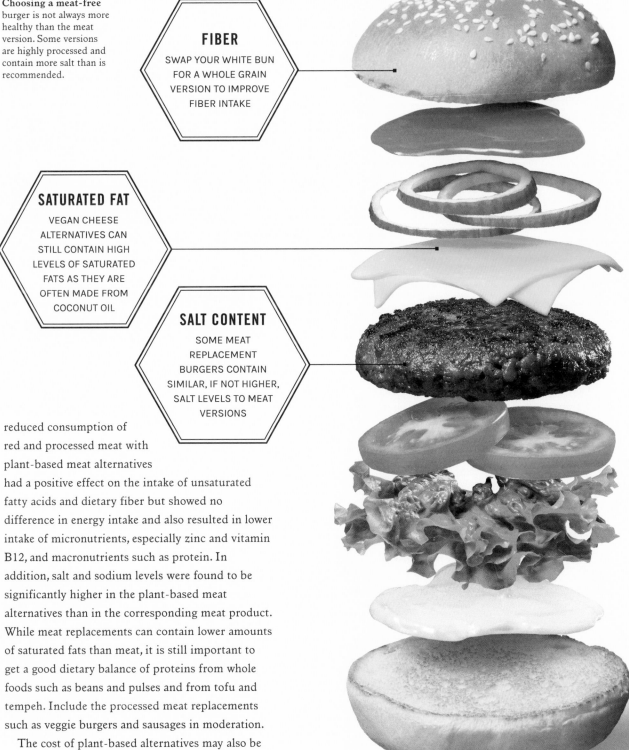

Choosing a meat-free burger is not always more healthy than the meat version. Some versions are highly processed and contain more salt than is recommended.

FIBER

SWAP YOUR WHITE BUN FOR A WHOLE GRAIN VERSION TO IMPROVE FIBER INTAKE

SATURATED FAT

VEGAN CHEESE ALTERNATIVES CAN STILL CONTAIN HIGH LEVELS OF SATURATED FATS AS THEY ARE OFTEN MADE FROM COCONUT OIL

SALT CONTENT

SOME MEAT REPLACEMENT BURGERS CONTAIN SIMILAR, IF NOT HIGHER, SALT LEVELS TO MEAT VERSIONS

reduced consumption of red and processed meat with plant-based meat alternatives had a positive effect on the intake of unsaturated fatty acids and dietary fiber but showed no difference in energy intake and also resulted in lower intake of micronutrients, especially zinc and vitamin B12, and macronutrients such as protein. In addition, salt and sodium levels were found to be significantly higher in the plant-based meat alternatives than in the corresponding meat product. While meat replacements can contain lower amounts of saturated fats than meat, it is still important to get a good dietary balance of proteins from whole foods such as beans and pulses and from tofu and tempeh. Include the processed meat replacements such as veggie burgers and sausages in moderation.

The cost of plant-based alternatives may also be a factor in day-to-day choices as they can be more expensive than the meat versions.

HOW SHOULD CHANGES IN DIET BE MANAGED?

Dietary changes should happen slowly and consistently. Instead of making drastic overnight changes, managing your body's adaptation to change over time is important to make sure you get the best results.

GRADUAL CHANGE

If you suddenly eat a lot of fiber from plants and whole grains in a way you haven't before, your body is likely to react. It takes the large intestine time to adjust to an increase in fiber because moving from a little to a lot can trigger our gut microbes to go into fermentation overdrive, resulting in more gas and bloating. To limit this, it is recommended to try and introduce one portion of extra fiber over a few days (see pp.80–81). For example, you could switch from white pasta to whole grain, then add lentils to your pasta sauce a few days later. A drastic overnight change may be possible for some people, but for most, embracing a plant-based diet while ensuring nutritional needs are met, requires time and careful planning. The large intestine needs time to adjust. Instead of making a sudden change, try a different way of starting the transition. That could be to have a meat-free day—one day a week without meat or dairy. After that, gradually build up the number of days a week you're meat-free. If you are going vegan and not just reducing animal products, then ensure you are taking the necessary supplements when you begin this transition (see pp.96–97).

HYDRATION

It is also important to consider hydration when changing your diet and adding fiber in particular. Fiber needs water so it can dissolve in the gut or be broken down by gut bacteria, and so you should aim to add an extra glass of water a day. Keep a bottle of water with you so that you can monitor your fluid intake. This will also help with bowel movements.

SEEK SUPPORT

Going at your own pace is important when making changes to your diet, and it is worth getting support from a health professional if you require advice. Arming yourself with recipes, changing your grocery shopping, and having a plan will help. Perhaps friends or family can be a part of this journey with you.

THINK ABOUT PLANT POINTS

Plant points have gained attention in recent years. Research shows that it is beneficial to our long-term health to include at least 30 types of plants in our diet over the course of a week (see pp.70–71). If you make this a habit, it is a useful way of getting more variety on your plate, more spices, herbs, pulses, vegetables, and fruits and flavors.

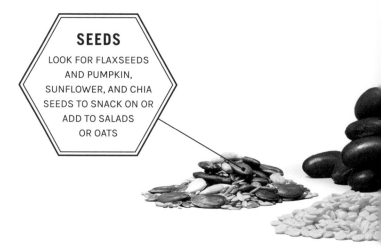

SEEDS

LOOK FOR FLAXSEEDS AND PUMPKIN, SUNFLOWER, AND CHIA SEEDS TO SNACK ON OR ADD TO SALADS OR OATS

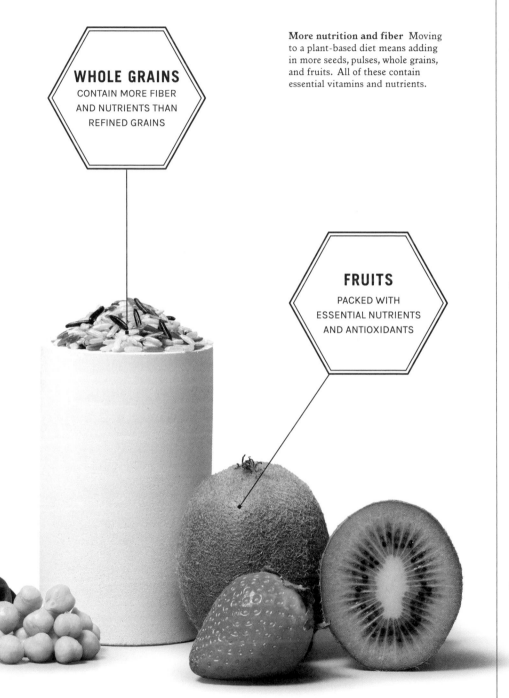

WHOLE GRAINS
CONTAIN MORE FIBER
AND NUTRIENTS THAN
REFINED GRAINS

More nutrition and fiber Moving
to a plant-based diet means adding
in more seeds, pulses, whole grains,
and fruits. All of these contain
essential vitamins and nutrients.

FRUITS
PACKED WITH
ESSENTIAL NUTRIENTS
AND ANTIOXIDANTS

Swaps to add more plant points

THERE ARE PLENTY OF WAYS
TO ADD MORE PLANTS TO
YOUR DIET. PLAN AHEAD AND
TRY THESE IDEAS TO GET YOUR
30 PLANT POINTS.

CARBOHYDRATES

SWAP WHITE CARBOHYDRATES
FOR WHOLE GRAINS—WHITE
BREAD TO WHOLE GRAIN
OR SEEDED

REDUCE MEAT

SLOWLY REDUCE MEAT—REPLACE
IT WITH LENTILS, BEANS, OR
PULSES IN FAMILY FAVORITES
SUCH AS LASAGNAS, STEWS,
AND BOLOGNESE

SNACKS

TRY NUTS OR FRUIT INSTEAD OF
CHIPS OR COOKIES TO SNACK
MORE HEALTHILY AND INCREASE
PLANT VARIETY

STOCK YOUR FREEZER

KEEP A STORE OF FROZEN
VEGETABLES AND FRUITS—THESE
OFTEN CONTAIN MORE NUTRITION
THAN THE FRESH VARIETY

SKINS

KEEP THE SKIN ON YOUR
VEGETABLES AND FRUITS—
TRY EATING THE SKIN WITH YOUR
KIWI FRUIT AND POTATOES

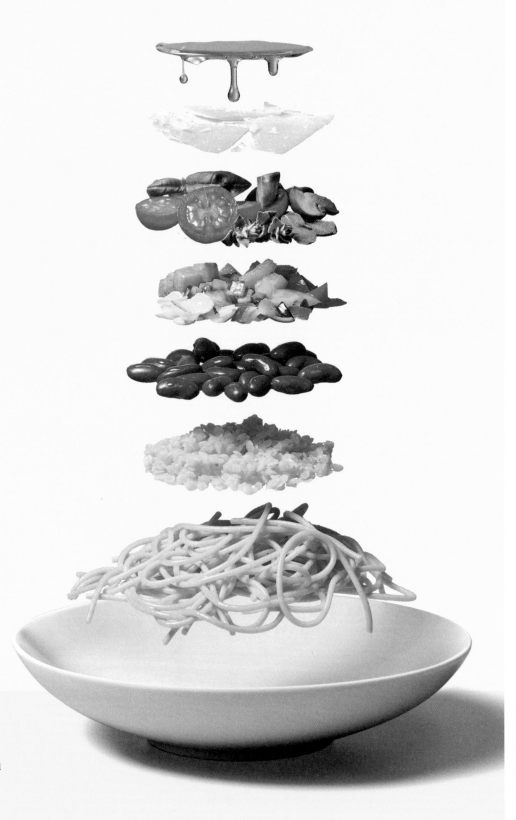

FATS

EXTRA-VIRGIN OLIVE
OIL, VEGAN PARMESAN
CHEESE OR NUTRITIONAL
YEAST (FORTIFIED WITH
VITAMIN B12)
ON TOP

VEGETABLES

COOKED TOMATOES
ARE RICH
IN NUTRIENTS,
INCLUDING A POWERFUL
ANTIOXIDANT
LYCOPENE

PROTEIN

KIDNEY BEANS AND
LENTILS ARE A GOOD
SOURCE OF PROTEIN
AND IRON,
WHEN PAIRED WITH
VITAMIN C

CARBS

WHOLE WHEAT
SPAGHETTI BOOSTS
FIBER INTAKE FOR YOUR
GUT MICROBES
TO ENJOY

Plant-based spaghetti bolognese
When eating plant-based, you can still
enjoy favorite family recipes by
swapping the red meat for beans and
lentils. This makes a nutritious meal and
is lower in fat than the classic version.

WHAT MIGHT A HEALTHY PLANT-BASED DIET LOOK LIKE?

As with all diets, what could be considered healthy will vary from person to person. As a general rule, a plant-based diet that is beneficial for your health should have the right quantity and quality of diverse food and contain lots of color.

A BALANCED PLATE

Healthy eating looks different for everyone. For some, adding a green vegetable or two each week is healthy, while for others reducing their sugar intake is beneficial. There is no single perfect, healthy diet that suits everyone. However, when striving to eat an optimal plant-based diet, there are a few useful guidelines. A balanced plate looks similar whether you are following a plant-based diet. It should include a source of carbohydrates (preferably whole grains), protein, vegetables, and healthy fats. Consumption of saturated/trans fats, sugar, salt, and red and processed meats should be low, while intake of fruits, vegetables, beans, and pulses should be high.

FISH

If you include fish in your diet (see pp.52–53), the recommendation for adults is to eat two portions of fish a week, one of which should be fatty (pilchards or salmon, for example). So this could include having a hake and couscous salad for lunch one day and a fillet of salmon along with a vegetable medley and potato wedges for dinner another day.

DAIRY AND EGGS

If you consume dairy foods (see pp.56–57), you can include them in your diet on a regular basis, as they provide vitamin B12, calcium, and iodine. A typical day with lots of calcium could include milk with overnight oats, tea, and coffee; plain yogurt; and small amounts of cheese. Cheese can be high in saturated fats and salt so keep consumption in moderation. Try to avoid high-sugar calcium-rich options, such as milkshakes or flavored yogurt. Read the labels and look for low-sugar options. Eggs are a highly nutritious addition to consume as part of a healthy diet. You could eat them hard-boiled as a snack, poached as part of a balanced breakfast with whole grain bread and tomatoes, or cooked in a vegetable frittata for lunch or dinner.

If you don't eat dairy, consume alternatives that are fortified or that naturally contain vitamin B12, calcium, and iodine. You might choose a plant-based fortified drink like almond, soy, or oat milk in place of cow's milk. A typical day following a diet avoiding dairy could include breakfast with a plant-based fortified drink such as overnight oats, teas and coffees with a fortified plant-based drink, a pasta bake containing vegetables, tofu for a source of calcium, topped with nutritional yeast for a source of vitamin B12 and a cheesy taste.

REDUCE RED AND PROCESSED MEATS

If you eat meat (see pp.58–59), reduce consumption of red and processed meats, read labels to avoid high fat and sugar content, and remove skin before cooking to lower the fat content. It is recommended to have no more than 2.5oz (70g) of cooked or processed red meat a day as it has been linked with bowel cancer. A diet containing meat could include a chicken salad for lunch and/or a turkey and vegetable curry with rice for dinner.

WHAT IF I ALSO EAT FISH?

Fish can be a healthy addition to a plant-based diet, if consumed in the right quantities, but sadly times are changing quickly and the quality of fish in the oceans is not as good as it once was.

If you are following a plant-based diet that involves fish, the advice is to eat at least 8oz of fish per week, including one of fatty fish. A typical serving is 5oz. Fish contains many beneficial nutrients such as vitamin B12, iodine, protein, and calcium in the bones and omega-3 in fatty fish. An analysis of 20 studies involving hundreds of thousands of participants indicated that eating approximately one to two 3oz servings of fatty fish a week—including salmon, herring, mackerel, anchovies, or sardines—

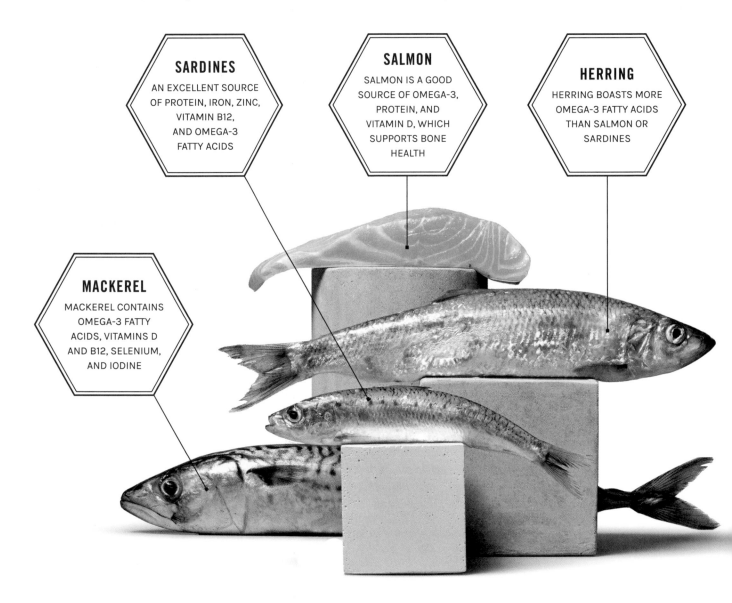

SARDINES
AN EXCELLENT SOURCE OF PROTEIN, IRON, ZINC, VITAMIN B12, AND OMEGA-3 FATTY ACIDS

SALMON
SALMON IS A GOOD SOURCE OF OMEGA-3, PROTEIN, AND VITAMIN D, WHICH SUPPORTS BONE HEALTH

HERRING
HERRING BOASTS MORE OMEGA-3 FATTY ACIDS THAN SALMON OR SARDINES

MACKEREL
MACKEREL CONTAINS OMEGA-3 FATTY ACIDS, VITAMINS D AND B12, SELENIUM, AND IODINE

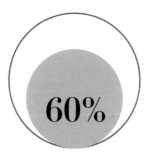

60%

OF GLOBAL FISH STOCKS
ARE FISHED TO
MAXIMUM
SUSTAINABLE YIELD

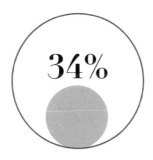

34%

OF STOCKS ARE BEING FISHED
BELOW THE BIOLOGICAL
SUSTAINABLE LEVELS. THIS MEANS
THAT A VIABLE POPULATION CANNOT
BE SUSTAINED AT THE CURRENT
LEVEL OF FISHING

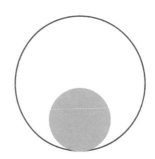

1/3 OF MONITORED
GLOBAL FISH STOCKS
ARE OVERFISHED

reduces the risk of dying from heart disease by 36 percent. Omega-3 may help reduce levels of fats called triglycerides in the blood, which are associated with a higher risk of cardiovascular disease. They are also believed to have anti-inflammatory properties that may help reduce hardening of the arteries. We also know that eating fatty fish reduces blood clotting and so can help cut the risk of stroke.

SEA POLLUTION

Although fish is a great source of nutrients, it can contain pollutants from the sea. In many parts of the world, there is a problem with chemical compounds known as polychlorinated biphenyls (PCBs), which were used in many industrial processes in the past and then leaked into the sea. Although these chemicals have been banned since 1979, they are often still found in the food chain, affecting many fish. The advice is to eat a range of fish and to remove the skin and cooking juices before eating.

CAN I CHOOSE SUSTAINABLE FISH?

It is now difficult to source sustainable fish. As sea temperatures rise and humans continue to pollute the oceans, sea life is left with low levels of dissolved oxygen, making it difficult to breathe. Today's assessment of wild Atlantic salmon populations in our rivers remains a serious cause for concern.

Although a great deal has already been done by environmental agencies, climate change, marine exploitation, and barriers to fish passage are all significantly impacting the numbers of salmon returning to our rivers to spawn.

WHAT ABOUT FARMED FISH?

Farmed fish accounts for more than half of the fish consumed globally, and aquaculture, or fish farming, is sometimes seen as a more sustainable option. But it comes with its own environmental issues. Some farming methods have negative impacts on the environment, and carnivorous species such as salmon and prawns require wild-caught fish in their die,t even if they themselves are farmed. If you wish to consume fish, the best thing you can do is to consume less and look for less common species to eat.

Children under 16

SOME FISH SHOULD BE AVOIDED BY CHILDREN AND PREGNANT WOMEN.

Children under the age of 16 should avoid eating any shark, swordfish, or marlin as the mercury in these fish can affect a child's nervous system. The same advice is also given to pregnant women as mercury can damage the fetus's nervous system.

WHAT IF I ALSO EAT EGGS?

Consuming eggs alongside a plant-based diet can be a helpful way of getting your key nutrients. Most of the nutrition from eggs is contained in the yolk.

A COMPLETE PROTEIN

Eggs are a complete protein, which means they contain all nine essential amino acids: histidine, isoleucine, leucine, lysine, methionine, phenylalanine, threonine, tryptophan, and valine. Eggs are considered one of the highest-quality forms of protein ahead of cow's milk and beef and have a significantly lower contribution to greenhouse gas emissions. Eggs contribute 1.8 percent of greenhouse gas emissions caused by dietary intake compared to red meat, which contributes 24.2 percent. Making a switch from meat to eggs may be a helpful plant-based dietary shift that is of benefit to the environment while still providing you with the nutrients you need for a healthy diet.

ARE EGGS HIGH IN CHOLESTEROL?

In the past, eggs have been incorrectly associated with raised cholesterol levels, which we now know to be incorrect. We used to think that cholesterol from foods like eggs caused higher blood cholesterol levels, but more recent research has shown that this cholesterol is far less harmful than the saturated fatty acids found in foods such as butter and fatty

meat like bacon. You may consume one egg a day as part of a healthy diet without increasing blood cholesterol levels.

ARE FREE-RANGE EGGS BETTER?

Some people prefer to buy free-range eggs due to concerns about animal welfare. Hens raised as free-range may have a little more space to move and have access to outdoor areas. Some studies suggest that their eggs may contain higher levels of omega-3 fatty acids and vitamin D, although this can vary, depending where the hen was raised. There may also be a lower environmental impact from free-range hens as they are not dependent on chicken feed and can forage for more natural food. Another factor for consumers may be the financial cost as free-range eggs are more expensive than other eggs.

Studies have shown that the age of the hens may have a greater effect on egg quality than whether they are free-range. It was found that free-range hens have a significantly higher shell weight. Another difference was that the yolk weight of the free-range eggs was significantly higher, although there was no difference for the egg white weight.

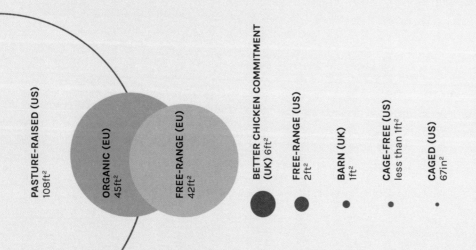

PASTURE-RAISED (US) 108ft² · ORGANIC (EU) 45ft² · FREE-RANGE (EU) 42ft² · BETTER CHICKEN COMMITMENT (UK) 6ft² · FREE-RANGE (US) 2ft² · BARN (UK) 1ft² · CAGE-FREE (US) less than 1ft² · CAGED (US) 67in²

HOW MUCH SPACE DO CHICKENS HAVE?

This graphic compares the areas provided per chicken under different farming systems. Most of the egg-laying hens in the US are raised in cages. Cage-free chickens are still very crowded with generally no outdoor access. Free-range hens have some outdoor time, and pasture-raised have the most outdoor space and best quality of life.

Egg labeling

THE WAY EGGS ARE LABELED VARIES FROM COUNTRY TO COUNTRY.
Look for information on the packaging for more information about egg welfare. In the US, there will be information from USDA Organic or other animal welfare organizations to make sure that the eggs meet humane and environmental standards. In the UK, the red lion mark shows that the egg meets regulated standards and is safe to eat.

NUTRIENTS
EGG YOLKS CONTAIN VITAMINS A, E, D, K, B. EGG YOLKS ARE A GOOD SOURCE OF PHOSPHORUS, ZINC, AND SELENIUM

EGG YOLKS
YOLKS ARE HIGH IN HEALTHY MONOUNSATURATED AND POLYUNSATURATED FATS, INCLUDING OMEGA-3 FATTY ACIDS

EGG WHITES
THESE CONTAIN NO FAT AND SMALLER AMOUNTS OF B VITAMINS AND MINERALS THAN THE YOLK

Vitamins and minerals for a whole egg

VITAMIN A 64mcg	**BIOTIN (B7)** 10mcg	**SELENIUM** 12mcg	**POTASSIUM** 73mg	**VITAMIN B6** 0.07mg
VITAMIN D 1.6mg	**VITAMIN B5** 0.7mg	**CALCIUM** 23mg	**ZINC** 0.6mg	**VITAMIN E** 0.7mg
RIBOFLAVIN (B2) 1.4mg	**CHOLINE** 144mg	**COPPER** 0.03mg	**OMEGA-3** 70mg	**VITAMIN K** 3.5mg
VITAMIN B12 1.4mg	**PHOSPHORUS** 91mg	**MAGNESIUM** 7mg	**THIAMINE (B1)** 0.04mg	
FOLATE (B9) 24mcg	**IODINE** 25mcg	**MANGANESE** 0.02mg	**NIACIN (B3)** 0.03mg	

WHAT IF I ALSO EAT DAIRY?

Consuming dairy is a personal decision. Ethically, using the milk from an animal that is meant to go to its young is difficult for many, and interestingly, more people choose to go dairy-free than meat-free. The nutritional benefits of dairy foods are, however, vast and heavily researched.

Including dairy in your plant-based diet can bring many nutritional advantages, although it may not suit everyone. Some research suggests that dairy is no longer considered the top source of calcium and protective factor for our bone health. Fortified foods such as plant-based milks and cereals are also great sources. A positive for many can be the inclusion of fermented dairy products (kefir, live yogurt, and traditional cheeses) to support a healthy gut microbiome. Some studies also show that higher intakes of dairy are associated with lower rates of type 2 diabetes, cardiovascular disease, improved weight management, and a lower risk of some cancers like colon cancer.

MILK AND HEALTH

Some people are concerned about the fat levels in milk and avoid it for that reason. However, studies have suggested that intake of high-fat dairy is not linked with obesity or cardiovascular disease. Advice in the past has been to include milk in your diet to keep your bones healthy as it has a high calcium content. However, a recent study of 200,000 women showed that milk intake was not linked with a reduction in hip fractures. As this is only one study and no men were included, it is hard to draw any definitive conclusions, but it may be supported by the fact that countries with high milk intakes, such as Scandinavia and the Netherlands, also have the highest fracture rates in the world.

ENVIRONMENTAL AND ANIMAL WELFARE CONCERNS

Making the switch to eating less or no dairy may benefit the environment. Although in the US, dairy contributes just 2 percent of greenhouse gas emissions, that is not the case for some countries. In the UK, dairy is the second-biggest contributor to greenhouse gas emissions after red meat at 14.3 percent, and it is estimated to be responsible for 11.7 percent of total dietary greenhouse gas emissions. Concerns about animal welfare are also behind many people's decision to cut dairy from their diet. Animal welfare and the separation of calves from their mothers so humans can drink their milk is something many struggle to accept. Opting for plant-based alternatives that are fortified with all the nutrients we need to be healthy is one way to help alleviate this problem.

If you are used to eating and drinking dairy products most days, you could make the change gradually, reducing dairy consumption to every other day then eventually to three days a week or less. To keep up your calcium intake, you can replace dairy milk and foods with plant-based alternatives that are fortified (this is often nonorganic) with calcium, vitamins B2, B12, D, and iodine (see pp.134–135). Organic products are sometimes not fortified, with a few exceptions, so check the labels to make sure. It is recommended that you speak to a health professional before you eliminate a whole food group to prevent deficiencies.

Dairy foods such as milk and cheese are a source of iodine, calcium, phosphorus, vitamin B12, and protein.

Lactose intolerance

WHILE MANY AVOID MILK AND DAIRY FOODS DUE TO ALLERGIES, THIS IS NOT A PROBLEM FOR THE VAST MAJORITY.

Some people cannot consume milk due to a lactose intolerance. This is due to a lack of lactase, the enzyme that breaks down lactose in the milk into more easily absorbable sugars. Many people have not evolved to process lactose effectively, and so it causes them problems, including bloating, stomach cramps, and diarrhea.

MILK
IF YOU DRINK MILK, TRY CUTTING DOWN FROM DAILY CONSUMPTION TO 2–3 DAYS A WEEK TO HELP THE PLANET

CHEESE
SOME CHEESES HAVE PROBIOTIC PROPERTIES THAT MAY BENEFIT GUT HEALTH AND CHOLESTEROL LEVELS

WHAT IF I ALSO EAT MEAT?

Whether someone chooses to eat meat is a personal choice made for health, animal welfare, or environmental reasons. However, if meat is something you choose to include in your diet, scientists and environmentalists recommend a reduction in the amount you consume both for your health and that of the planet.

WHY EAT MEAT?

It is possible to still eat meat while following a plant-based diet, although it is worth being aware of the impact of this both on your health and on the environment. Red meat (beef, lamb, pork, and venison) is a rich source of protein (see pp.20–21), vitamins B12, B6, B3, vitamin D, iron, zinc, and phosphorus, as well as long-chain omega-3 polyunsaturated fats, riboflavin, pantothenic acid, and selenium. Poultry (chicken, turkey, duck, and goose) also contains complete protein, vitamins B2, B3, B6, B12, zinc, and selenium. If you want to include some meat in your diet, the recommendation for each person is to have no more than 2.5oz (70g) a day or 12–18oz (350–500g) per week. Where possible, avoid eating too many processed meats such as sausages, ham, salami, and bacon because they are linked with a higher rate of bowel cancer (see pp.188–189).

PRODUCTION AND CONSUMPTION

The world now produces more than four times the quantity of meat than 50 years ago—from around 83 million tons in 1961 to 375 million tons in 2018. The average person in the world consumed around 51lb (23kg) of meat in 1961 compared with 95lb (43kg) in

Comparison of different meats

When choosing which meat to eat, consider the nutritional values for the type of meat per 3.5oz (100g) as well as their environmental impact. You can also take into account where the meat has come from, choosing local sources and high welfare farms where possible.

CHICKEN

CALORIES: **165**
PROTEIN: **31.02g**
FAT: **6.5g**
SATURATED FAT: **1.01g**

These figures are based on a 3.5oz (100g) portion of skinless, boneless chicken breast. Chicken with skin will have higher fat values.

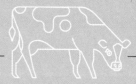

BEEF

CALORIES: **217**
PROTEIN: **26.1g**
FAT: **11.8g**
SATURATED FAT: **6g**

Based on a 3.5oz (100g) serving of ground beef with 10% fat content. Choose lean cuts and avoid processed beef where possible.

2014. This ranges from more than 220lb (100kg) per person in the US and Australia to the lowest amount of 11lb (5kg) in India. Currently in the US, more than 86 percent of the population eats meat.

ENVIRONMENTAL IMPACT

The impact of meat consumption on the environment is vast. Off all the animal species, cattle are responsible for the most emissions, representing about 65 percent of the livestock sector's emissions. About 44 percent of livestock emissions are in the form of methane (CH_4). The remaining part is almost equally shared between nitrous oxide (N_2O; 29 percent) and carbon dioxide (CO_2; 27 percent). Methane is 80 times more potent at warming than carbon dioxide as a greenhouse gas—it has accounted for roughly 30 percent of global warming since preindustrial times, and it is a primary contributor to the formation of the ground level ozone layer

Enteric fermentation is a part of the digestive process in animals such as cattle, sheep, and buffalo, which produces methane as a by-product. Therefore, if we all can take responsibility and cut our meat consumption, it will help the environment.

Cutting down

YOU CAN CUT DOWN ON RED AND PROCESSED MEAT BY EATING SMALLER PORTIONS LESS OFTEN. THE FOLLOWING SWAPS COULD HELP:

- **Ground** swap ground lamb or beef for turkey or vegetarian options
- **Sandwiches** swap one of your ham or beef sandwiches for a non-red meat filling such as chicken or fish
- **Burger** Swap your quarter pound burger for a standard burger or you could choose a chicken, fish, or veggie burger instead
- **Sausages** Have two pork sausages rather than three, and add a portion of vegetables. Opt for reduced-fat sausages
- **Steak** Swap an 8oz (163g) steak for a 5oz (102g) version
- **Stews** Swap the meat in stews, casseroles, and curries for vegetables, beans, pulses, mushrooms, and tofu

Try to have a meat-free day each week. Swap red or processed meat for beans, lentils, and veggies. Eventually, swapping meat for plant proteins will have a huge impact on the environment.

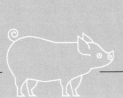

PORK

CALORIES: **242**
PROTEIN: **27g**
FAT: **14g**
SATURATED FAT: **5g**

Choose lean cuts such as tenderloin or loin over pork belly or processed versions. Try baking or grilling rather than frying.

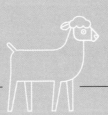

LAMB

CALORIES: **294**
PROTEIN: **25g**
FAT: **21g**
SATURATED FAT: **9g**

Lamb is relatively high in saturated fat so look for lean cuts and be aware of healthy portion sizes.

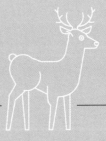

VENISON

CALORIES: **158**
PROTEIN: **30g**
FAT: **3.1g**
SATURATED FAT: **1.3g**

Venison is a lean meat that is lower in fat (especially saturated fat) than most other meats. Wild venison may have different values from farm-grown.

IS PLANT-BASED PROCESSED FOOD HEALTHIER?

Regardless of whether a food is plant-based, if an item is ultra-processed, it is likely to not be the best choice. Understanding the difference between processed and ultra-processed foods will help you make the right decisions for your long-term health.

WHAT IS PROCESSED FOOD?

Scientists have been debating the way we process foods for a long time, and most conclude that food processing in itself is not the issue. Most of the food we eat today is processed in some way—for example, chickpeas in a can or vegetables that are chopped and put into bags are processed foods. However, these are minimally processed in a way that allows them to be stored or safer to eat. Some processing methods, such as fermentation, have been around for thousands of years and are beneficial for our health (see pp.76–77).

ULTRA-PROCESSED FOODS

While some processed foods are not bad for you, one group known as ultra-processed foods (UPFs), sometimes called junk or fast food, is less healthy. UPFs are snacks, drinks, ready-made meals, and many other food types formulated mostly or entirely from substances extracted from foods or derived from food constituents. They are made from ingredients that are processed, such as vegetable oils, flours, whey proteins, and sugars, and then often have additives and flavorings added to improve their taste and shelf life. It is these items, regardless of whether they are plant-based, that are less healthy choices than unprocessed or minimally processed foods. UPFs tend to be low in fiber and high in sugar, salt, and fat compared with less processed foods.

PLANT-BASED PROCESSED FOODS

Plant-based processed foods include meat substitutes to replace items like nuggets, sausage, and burgers. There is often a perception that plant-based processed foods are healthier than other UPFs as a plant-based

NOVA food classification

NOVA is a food classification system that classifies all foods into four groups, depending on how processed these items are. It can be a useful guide to the types of food we consume, although there are some concerns with its oversimplification. For example, soy foods are classed as ultra-processed, even though they have many nutrients and benefits.

UNPROCESSED OR MINIMALLY PROCESSED FOODS

LEGUMES, VEGETABLES, FRUITS, STARCHY ROOTS AND TUBERS, GRAINS, NUTS, BEEF, EGGS, CHICKEN, MILK

These foods are in their natural state without any substances being added. Inedible parts may be removed.

diet is associated with positive health outcomes. This is not the case because these products can often contain more fat, sugar, and salt than meat and just as much as other processed foods made from animal products. Always read the labels to find the salt and fat levels and to check for preservatives and additives. So much of our food is now ultra-processed that it is hard to avoid, and many are safe to eat as long as they do not make up the majority of you diet. It is the overconsumption of these foods that has led to an increase in obesity and many associated health issues.

Wherever possible, try to get most of your nutrition from unprocessed foods in their natural state, and prepare meals using fresh ingredients. In so doing you are drawing on the health benefits of something called the "food matrix", which refers to the various physical and chemical interactions between compounds present in food, and comprises over 150,000 components potentially beneficial to health. In manufacturing UPFs we deconstruct this matrix and so lose these benefits.

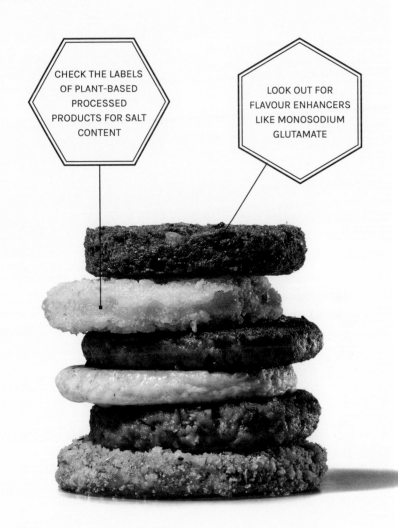

CHECK THE LABELS OF PLANT-BASED PROCESSED PRODUCTS FOR SALT CONTENT

LOOK OUT FOR FLAVOUR ENHANCERS LIKE MONOSODIUM GLUTAMATE

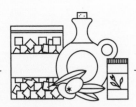

PROCESSED CULINARY INGREDIENTS

SALT, SUGAR, PLANT OILS, BUTTER, CREAM, HONEY, SALT

These are whole foods that have been processed minimally through pressing, refining, grinding, milling, and drying.

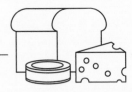

PROCESSED FOODS

BOTTLED VEGETABLES, MEAT IN SALT SOLUTION, FRUIT IN SYRUP OR CANDIED, BREAD, CHEESES, PUREES, PASTES

These foods are unprocessed or minimally processed foods before salt, oil, or sugar is added, and they are canned, pickled, smoked, or fermented.

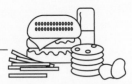

ULTRA-PROCESSED FOODS

COOKIES, ICE CREAM, READY-MADE MEALS, SOFT DRINKS, HAMBURGERS, NUGGETS

This group of food contains products made from a number of industrial processes such as extraction and chemical modification.

SHOULD I STILL AIM FOR LOW FAT?

There is now more awareness that not all fat is bad but still confusion around which types to include in the diet and those to avoid.

Fat is an essential part of your diet, although you need to be aware of the different kinds of fats are some are better than others. Generally, we need to cut down on saturated and trans fats and eat foods containing polyunsaturated and monounsaturated fats, and unsaturated fatty acids (see pp.20–21). Plant foods are naturally lower in saturated fats and trans fats than meat and dairy foods. Healthy fats shouldn't be avoided and are important for our enjoyment of food due to the role of fat in flavor, texture, mouthfeel, and satiety, as well as providing important nutrients. Some countries have a color labeling system showing at a glance whether a food is healthy. However, some foods that contain high levels of monounsaturated "good fats," such as olive oil, may be categorized as high in fat, so this system has limitations. The US FDA has strict guidelines around labeling what can be called "low" or "high" depending on percent daily value (%DV).

CHECK THE LABEL

If you are trying to reduce fat intake, buying the food with "low fat" on the label is not always the best option. Often these products contain sugar,

Food labels

Many countries use a system like this on food labels. Foods are categorized using green, yellow, and red lights to indicate low, medium, or high in sugar, salt, and fat. RIs are recommended intakes.

LOW	MEDIUM	HIGH (> 25% RIs)
Food with a green light is low in salt, fat, and sugar and is a healthy choice.	Food with a yellow light is neither high nor low in a nutrient and can be eaten most of the time.	Red light foods are high in salt, fat, or sugar. Try to eat less of these.
FAT < 3g/100g	FAT 3–7.5g/100g	FAT up to 17.5g/100g
SATURATED FAT < 1.5g/100g	SATURATED FAT 1.5–5g/100g	SATURATED FAT up to 5.0g/100g
SUGARS (TOTAL) < 5g/100g	SUGARS (TOTAL) 5–20g/100g	SUGARS (TOTAL) up to 22.5g/100g
SALT < 0.3g/100g	SALT 0.5–1.3g/100g	SALT up to 1.5g/100g

Percent daily value

NUTRITION LABELS IN THE US USE %DV (PERCENT DAILY VALUE) TO DETERMINE WHETHER A SERVING OF FOOD IS HIGH OR LOW IN A NUTRIENT. You can use percent daily values to make informed choices when buying food. As a general guide, 5% DV or less of a nutrient per serving is considered low; 20% DV or more of a nutrient per serving is considered high. Look for foods that are higher in dietary fiber, vitamin D, calcium, iron, and potassium and lower in saturated fat, sodium, and added sugars. When comparing foods, make sure that you're comparing the same serving sizes and use %DV to balance your intake through the day. Trans fats and proteins have no percentage values so use the number of grams as a guide.

Healthy plant fats These are some plant foods that contain monounsaturated fat as well as many other healthy nutrients. Eating them as part of a balanced diet will help you get the fats you need to stay healthy.

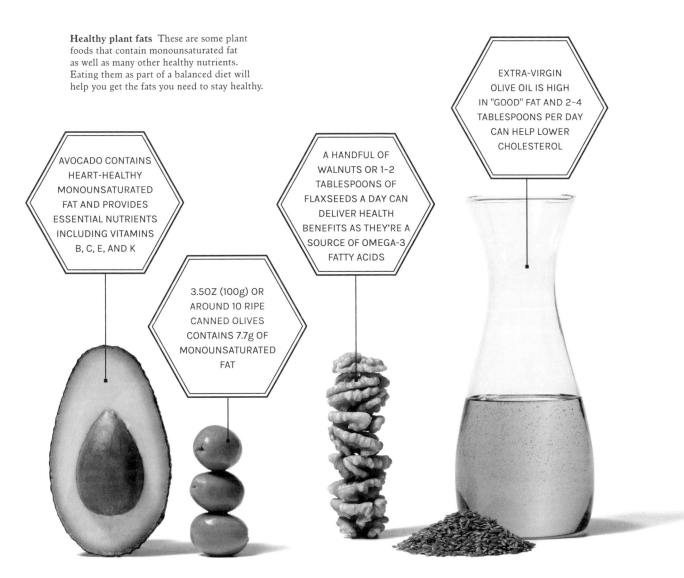

EXTRA-VIRGIN OLIVE OIL IS HIGH IN "GOOD" FAT AND 2–4 TABLESPOONS PER DAY CAN HELP LOWER CHOLESTEROL

AVOCADO CONTAINS HEART-HEALTHY MONOUNSATURATED FAT AND PROVIDES ESSENTIAL NUTRIENTS INCLUDING VITAMINS B, C, E, AND K

A HANDFUL OF WALNUTS OR 1–2 TABLESPOONS OF FLAXSEEDS A DAY CAN DELIVER HEALTH BENEFITS AS THEY'RE A SOURCE OF OMEGA-3 FATTY ACIDS

3.5OZ (100g) OR AROUND 10 RIPE CANNED OLIVES CONTAINS 7.7g OF MONOUNSATURATED FAT

which the body lays down as fat if eaten to excess, as well as other ingredients to improve their flavoring. Excess sugar, sugar-free substitutes like aspartame, and artificial additives are more harmful than moderate fat intake. It is better to get the fat your body needs from natural products, such as nuts, seeds, fish, and olive oil.

WHICH FATS TO AVOID

The World Health Organization recommends that intake of saturated fats should be no more than 10 percent of our total energy intake (TEI) and trans fats should make up no more than 1 percent of our TEI. Trans fats have been removed from many store-bought foods, but some baked goods may still include them. Check for trans fat by looking for hydrogenated oil on the label.

WHICH FATS SHOULD I CHOOSE?

Healthy fats are polyunsaturated, found in sunflower, soy, corn, and sesame oils and spreads, or monounsaturated, such as in olive and canola oils and spreads. If you include unsaturated fatty acids in foods in your diet, such as olive oil, avocados, nuts, seeds, and olives, they can improve cholesterol levels and help the absorption of vitamins A, D, E, and K.

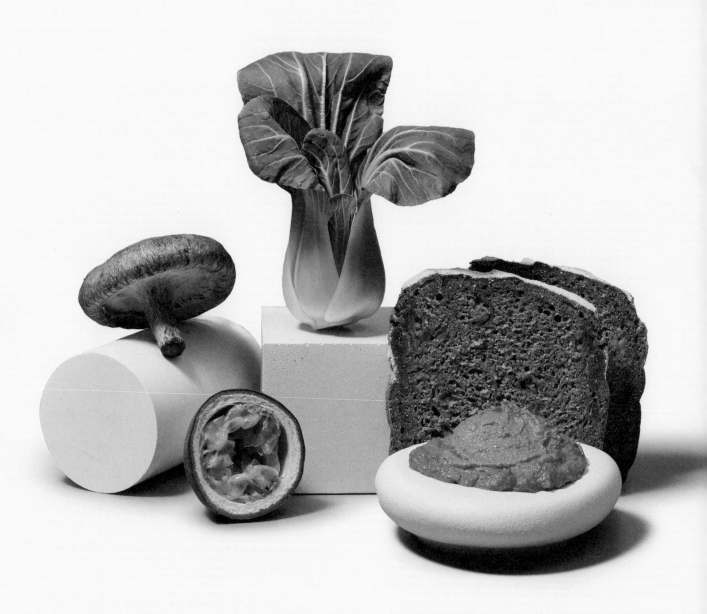

PLANT DIVERSITY

WHY IS IT IMPORTANT TO INCREASE PLANT DIVERSITY?

Eating a variety of plant foods helps maintain a healthy body in several ways, including supporting the microbes inside our gut known as the gut microbiota.

Eating a variety of plants has been demonstrated as crucial for our overall health and well-being because plants contain nutrients we simply cannot get in abundance from other foods. Fiber, vitamins, minerals, phytochemicals, and antioxidants from plants keep our bodies functioning well and our immune systems supported. Sadly, today's world doesn't celebrate the diversity of plants, with shoppers conditioned to purchase from a narrow range of options.

Eating a range of plant foods helps promote a more diverse growth of healthy bacteria, leading to a healthy microbiome, more SCFAs, and better overall health.

FIBER AND GUT HEALTH

Fibers are forms of carbohydrates that cannot be broken down by the small intestine and reach the large intestine intact, where they are fermented by gut bacteria or "microbiota." These microbiota need the indigestible plant fiber we consume to produce short-chain fatty acids (SCFAs) such as butyrate, which have many

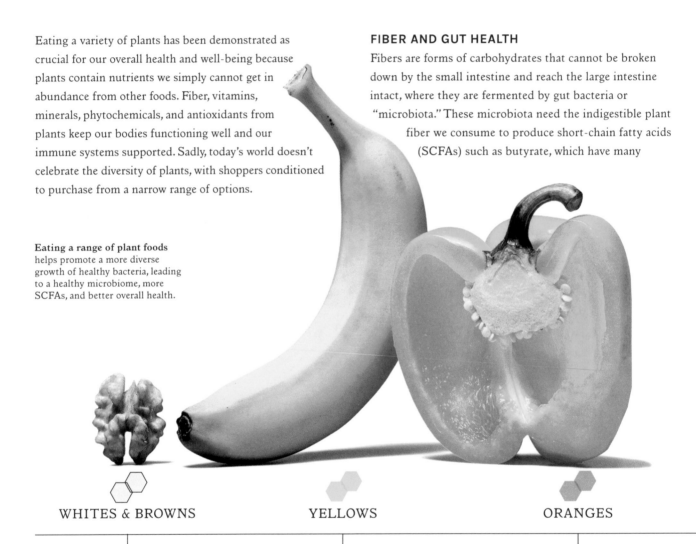

WHITES & BROWNS

Paler, fiber-rich foods typically benefit from lignans with antioxidants, which may help protect against ailments and cell damage.

NUTS | SEEDS | GRAINS | LENTILS
MUSHROOMS | CAULIFLOWER

YELLOWS

These tend to be rich in vitamin C, which helps protect cells, maintain healthy skin and bones, and has a role in wound healing.

BANANAS | GRAPEFRUIT | LEMONS
PINEAPPLE | PLANTAINS | POTATOES
SUMMER SQUASH | CORN

ORANGES

The body turns orange beta-carotene into vitamin A, linked to immunity and eye health, and essential for growth.

APRICOTS | CARROTS | MANGOES
ORANGES | PERSIMMONS | PUMPKINS
SWEET POTATOES

benefits, including promoting the health of colon cells. There is strong evidence that diets rich in fiber, particularly cereal fiber and whole grains, are associated with a lower risk of many health conditions, including cardiovascular disease, heart disease, stroke, type 2 diabetes, and colorectal cancer. We now know that there may be hundreds of different types of fibers that our bodies are designed to consume, and by increasing plant diversity, we increase the variety of fibers in our diet, bringing many health benefits (see pp.74–75).

ONLY 12 PLANT SPECIES AND 5 ANIMAL SPECIES ACCOUNT FOR 75 PERCENT OF THE WORLD'S FOOD PRODUCTION

A RANGE OF ANTIOXIDANTS

Nutrient antioxidants, such as vitamins A, C, and E and the minerals copper, zinc, and selenium, work by neutralizing "free radicals," molecules harmful to the body and linked to a number of diseases. In order to get a variety of nutrient

antioxidants, it is important to consume lots of different colorful plants as each color often gives a different nutritional component and antioxidant (see pp.86–87).

BIOAVAILABILITY

Consuming a wide variety of plant foods also enables us to maximize the absorption of nutrients in our bodies. For example, when consuming iron-rich pulses alongside the vitamin C found in tomatoes, we absorb more iron. Some plants, such as whole grains and beans, also contain phytates, which can reduce zinc absorption (see pp.88–91). By seeking out variety in a plant-based diet, and trying to avoid eating the same foods day in day out, we can help meet our nutritional requirements with a food-first approach, before considering nutritional supplements that can often be required on a plant-based diet (see pp.96–97).

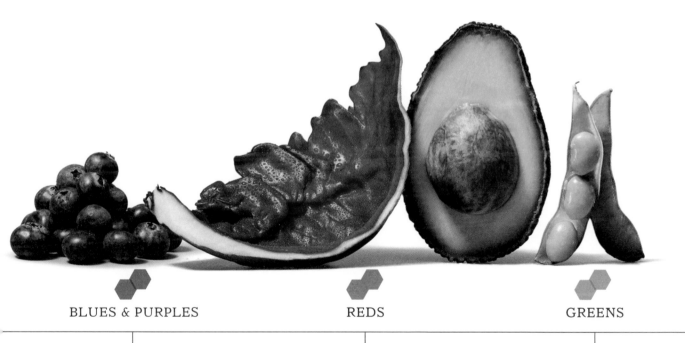

BLUES & PURPLES — REDS — GREENS

Resveratrol is a powerful antioxidant that helps protect blood vessels and is found in many blue and purple foods.

ACAI | BEETS | BLACKBERRIES BLACK CURRANTS | BLUEBERRIES | GRAPES EGGPLANT | FIGS | OLIVES | PLUMS PURPLE CARROTS | RAISINS | TARO

Red plants tend to contain potassium, which helps with healthy blood pressure

RED CABBAGE | TOMATOES | RADISHES RADICCHIO | STRAWBERRIES WATERMELON | RASPBERRIES CHERRIES | POMEGRANATES

Green foods are the main source of vitamin K for vegans, vital for blood clotting and bone health.

ASPARAGUS | AVOCADOS | BROCCOLI BRUSSELS SPROUTS | CABBAGE | CELERY FENNEL | GREEN BEANS | HERBS | KALE BOK CHOY | PEAS | PEPPERS | SPINACH

HOW DOES PLANT DIVERSITY SUPPORT GUT HEALTH?

We know that eating a variety of plant foods helps us increase fiber content in our diets, which, in turn, improves the microbiome of our gut.

EATING A VARIETY OF PLANTS

Aiming to get a large variety of different plant foods in the diet—not just fruits and vegetables but also nuts and seeds, legumes, whole grains, and herbs and spices—helps our gut microbiota thrive (see pp.66–67). This results in plenty of good gut bacteria that are able to perform their day-to-day tasks efficiently.

When we have a good, diverse array of gut microbes provided by a diverse diet, they can provide many benefits to our health—for example, supporting our immune system,

protecting our gut barrier, helping maintain normal blood sugar levels, communicating messages to the brain from our gut and vice versa, and producing essential hormones and neurotransmitters such as serotonin.

THE ROLE OF PHYTOCHEMICALS

Phytochemicals are organic compounds found in plant foods. A recent review suggested that phytochemicals entering the intestinal ecosystem can alter the composition of microbial ecology beneficially by acting as prebiotics and antimicrobial agents against harmful gut microbiota.

Prebiotics are dietary fibres that feed beneficial gut bacteria (see pp.16–17), which helps maintain a healthy gut microbiome.

Phytochemicals may also help reduce the risk of gut disorders and colorectal cancer and help modulate gut hormones. Resveratrol is a phytochemical found in red grapes and blueberries and is linked to health benefits. It is the compound that gives these foods their color and has antioxidant and anti-inflammatory properties that may have positive benefits for cardiovascular disease, neurodegenerative disorders, cancer, and obesity.

> BLUEBERRIES, SPINACH, AND TOMATOES ALL CONTAIN POLYPHENOLS, WHICH ARE IMPORTANT FOR GUT HEALTH

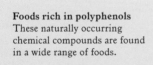

Foods rich in polyphenols
These naturally occurring chemical compounds are found in a wide range of foods.

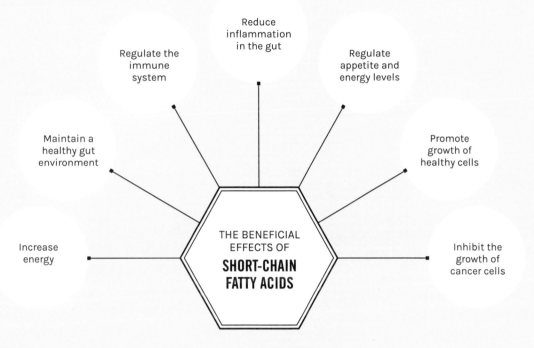

Reduce inflammation in the gut

Regulate the immune system

Regulate appetite and energy levels

Maintain a healthy gut environment

Promote growth of healthy cells

Increase energy

THE BENEFICIAL EFFECTS OF **SHORT-CHAIN FATTY ACIDS**

Inhibit the growth of cancer cells

DO POLYPHENOLS HELP GUT HEALTH?

Polyphenols are one diverse group of phytochemicals found in plant foods such as spinach, broccoli, tomatoes, and dark berries like blueberries. Around 90 percent of polyphenols are absorbed by the body, and the remaining amount are fed to our gut microbes in the large intestines. This is where they begin to have beneficial properties for our bodies. Some have have been shown to increase specific strains of bacteria, such as *Bifidobacterium* and *Lactobacillus,* which we use in a lot of food items and which can help prevent disease and provide anti-inflammatory effects and cardiovascular protection. You will notice these particular strains are often found in yogurts. By eating a varied and balanced diet, you will get a range of polyphenols.

FERMENTATION AND SHORT-CHAIN FATTY ACIDS

Increased fiber from eating more plant-based foods such as fruits, vegetables, and whole grains can support our gut health as it helps the body produce more bacteria in the gut. Undigested fiber reaches the colon where it ferments or is eaten by the bacteria in the gut and releases compounds called short-chain-fatty acids, or SFCAs. These SFCAs have highly beneficial properties. The most researched SFCA, butyrate, is associated with multiple health benefits such as improved sleep, decreased inflammation, and decreased risk of colon cancer. Others, such as acetate and propionate, also may have benefits that we are not yet fully aware of, including positive effects on brain functioning.

WHAT ARE PLANT POINTS AND WHY 30?

We know that eating a variety of plant-based foods is beneficial. Eating 30 different plant types a week can actively support your gut microbiome, and using plant points can help you keep track of how much variety you're eating.

Unlike the "5 A Day" campaigns that tend to target only our consumption of fruits and vegetables, plant points recognize the importance of all plant-derived ingredients. In this context, a plant is any kind of food that has been grown—not only fruits and vegetables but also grains, beans and pulses, nuts and seeds, and even herbs and spices.

GARDENING FOR THE GUT

Each strain of bacteria in your gut needs different types of plant foods to function effectively and help keep your body energized and healthy (see pp.68–69). Hence, eating a wide range of plants helps cultivate a varied and flourishing garden of beneficial

RESEARCH INDICATES EATING ACROSS THE SUPER SIX CAN ADD UP TO A DECADE OF HEALTHY YEARS TO YOUR LIFE

bacteria in the gut. Recent research discovered that people who frequently consume 30 or more different types of plant foods a week had a significantly more diverse gut microbiome than those eating 10 or fewer. Those eating a wider variety of plants have also been found to harbor a greater proportion of the bacteria that produce beneficial compounds called short-chain fatty acids (SCFAs), which may reduce the risk of inflammatory diseases, type 2 diabetes, obesity, heart disease, and other conditions (see pp.68–69).

KEEPING COUNT

One way to make sure that you're getting a variety of plant types in your diet is to count plant points over the course of a week. Many people struggle to reach their 5-a-day and may feel daunted at the prospect of 30. However, once you understand the six plant food groups that count toward your total, it will feel much simpler to achieve. There are numerous ideas for how to achieve 30 plant points on pp.72–73.

Six plant food groups known as the Super Six are counted for plant points. These are vegetables, fruits, whole grains, legumes (beans and pulses), nuts and seeds, and herbs and spices.

Do go gentle

UPPING PLANT-BASED VARIETY INCREASES FIBER IN THE DIET, WHICH CAN LEAD TO MORE GAS, BLOATING, DIARRHEA, AND CONSTIPATION.
Here are some simple tips to reduce discomfort:

Start slowly: add one new food at a time and try adding another only once your body has adapted.
Stay hydrated: fluid levels are important to support digestion and keep food and waste moving through.
Keep moving: stretching exercises and yoga help strengthen the muscles used during digestion and aid with the process of digestion too.
Sit up and chew: sitting up straight helps with the flow of food through the body, and chewing food well ensures it reaches the stomach ready to be digested.

Eating for your gut bacteria
Eating the widest variety of plants helps support a diversity of beneficial gut bacteria, which studies increasingly show are vital to many aspects of health, from immune response to cognition and even mood.

What are the Super Six?

Research indicates that people who consume high-fiber diets made up of a wide range of whole plant-based foods from the "Super Six" typically have the greatest gut microbiome.

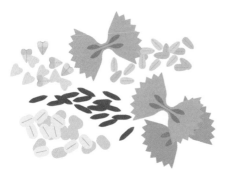

WHOLE GRAINS
1 point

EXAMPLES

oats, whole wheat pasta, spelt, buckwheat, quinoa, red rice

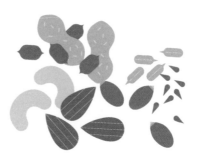

NUTS AND SEEDS
1 point

EXAMPLES

walnuts, cashews, peanuts, almonds, chai seeds, pumpkin seeds, sunflower seeds, hemp seeds, flaxseeds

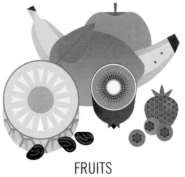

FRUITS
1 point

EXAMPLES

apples, bananas, berries, mango, pineapple, kiwi, pears, dates, raisins

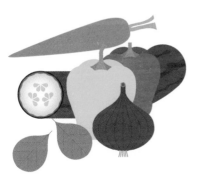

VEGETABLES
1 point

EXAMPLES

carrots, broccoli, kale, spinach, cucumber, radishes, peppers, mushrooms, onions

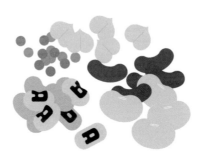

LEGUMES
1 point

EXAMPLES

lentils, chickpeas, kidney beans, black-eyed peas, cannellini beans

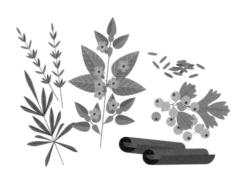

HERBS AND SPICES
¼ point

EXAMPLES

oregano, thyme, rosemary, cilantro, turmeric, cayenne pepper, paprika, cumin, cinnamon

HOW CAN I INCREASE THE DIVERSITY OF PLANTS I EAT?

Many of us struggle to eat the 5-a-day recommendation of fruits and vegetables, so achieving 30 plant points a week may seem a little overwhelming. Here are some helpful pointers to get you started.

FILL YOUR PLATE WELL

When planning your meals, use these ideas to get a variety of plant foods through the week. Once you get used to eating this way, it will become a habit.

● **Fill half of your plate with vegetables.** Include plenty of colors on your plate and enjoy vegetables as a snack with hummus, salsa, or guacamole.

● **Change the way you think about meat.** Have smaller amounts. Use it as a garnish instead of a centerpiece.

● **Choose good fats.** Fats in olive oil, olives, nuts and nut butters, seeds, and avocados are particularly healthy choices.

● **Eat vegetarian at least one night a week.** Build the meals around beans, whole grains, and vegetables.

● **Include whole grains for breakfast.** Start with oatmeal, quinoa, buckwheat, or barley. Then add some nuts or seeds along with fresh fruit.

● **Go for greens.** Try a variety of green leafy vegetables such as kale, Swiss chard, spinach, and other greens each day. Steam, grill, braise, or stir-fry to preserve their flavor and nutrients.

● **Build a meal around a salad.** Fill a bowl with salad greens such as romaine, spinach, butter lettuce, and/or spicier salads like arugula, watercress, or mustard greens. Add an assortment of other vegetables along with fresh herbs, beans, peas, tofu, tempeh, or mycoprotein (see pp.122–123).

● **Eat fruit for dessert.** A ripe, juicy peach; a refreshing slice of watermelon; or a crisp apple will satisfy your craving for a sweet bite after a meal.

Organize your kitchen

TRY SOME OF THESE IDEAS TO EAT A DIVERSE RANGE OF FOODS

Ordering veggie boxes encourages diversity as they usually include a large variety of colorful and seasonal vegetables. They may also be good value for money for fresh fruits and veggies every week.

Pack your freezer full of frozen plant foods such as fruits, like berries or bananas, and veggies, such as peas or spinach.

Try adding fermented foods, including kombucha, kefir, sauerkraut, and kimchi to your plate.

Opt for a mixed bag of salad rather than a single type.

Choose different colors of the same vegetable.

MAKE CHANGE SLOWLY

If you are new to eating a plant-based diet, a good way to start building your meals is to try out the 1, 2, 3 guide. This model suggests that when building your plant-based plate, try adding 1 whole grain, 2 nuts or seeds, and 3 fruits and vegetables. For those who struggle with vegetables, try slowly adding meat-free days every week and bulk up your usual dishes with beans and pulses. You can also try including "hidden" greens and veggies into foods such as pasta sauces. These can include spinach, kale, or Swiss chard, which you can blend first or cook to break down into small pieces in a sauce.

Mixed beans
These store pantry essentials are nutritious and high in protein, fiber, iron, and B vitamins.

AFFORDABLE

Grains
Try quinoa, bulgur wheat, whole wheat pasta, or brown rice with sauces, soups, and salads.

WHOLE GRAIN

Mixed leaves
Include 3–4 types of leaves (for example, spinach, arugula, and lettuce) to increase your plant points.

VARIETY

Soups
Add your favorite veggies, beans, grains, herbs, and spices to make a delicious, plant-powered meal!

VERSATILE

Mixed nuts and seeds
Add to breakfast oat bowls, smoothies, soups, salads, or yogurt.

CRUNCH

Smoothies
Make using fresh or frozen fruits or veggies. You can also add in seeds and nuts for extra plant points.

EXTRA POINTS

Spices
Using spices adds instant flavor as well as extra plant points and important antioxidants to a meal.

FLAVOR

Fruit
Try frozen or canned fruits to build up the range of foods you're eating throughout the year.

SWEET

Berries
Fresh or frozen, these are packed full of essential nutrients such as vitamins, minerals, and antioxidants.

NUTRIENTS

Herbs
Add fresh, dried, or frozen herbs to increase depth and flavor of a range of dishes and add plant points.

SPICES

Fermented
Eat yogurt containing active cultures or add sauerkraut to salads to get fermented foods into your diet.

GUT HEALTH

Opt for these items

A range of food types can help you add more plant types into your weekly diet. Use some of these tips to help you get as many different types as possible.

WHY IS IT SO IMPORTANT TO GET ENOUGH FIBER?

Consuming fiber has been linked to many positive health benefits, including improved heart and colon health. Fiber intake may even affect our life span, but most of us are still eating only half of the recommended 30g a day.

WHAT IS FIBER?

Fiber is a type of carbohydrate that is found only in plant foods. Our bodies cannot break it down efficiently using digestive enzymes, and so our gut microbiome metabolizes the fiber into short-chain fatty acids (SCFAs). It used to be thought that fiber had no benefit as we could not break it down in our bodies, but we now understand just how vitally important it is. There is strong evidence that diets rich in fiber, particularly whole grain fiber (found in whole wheat bread, whole wheat pasta, brown rice, oats, quinoa, and barley, for example), are associated with a lower risk of many health conditions, including heart disease such as angina and heart attacks, stroke, type 2 diabetes, and colon cancer.

There are two main types of fiber—soluble and insoluble—although many foods contain both types.

SOLUBLE FIBER

Soluble fiber dissolves in water and turns to gel during digestion, slowing the digestive process, which helps keep blood sugar levels stable (see pp.172–173). It is found in foods such as oats, nuts, seeds, lentils, peas, beans, and some fruits and vegetables.

INSOLUBLE FIBER

Insoluble fiber does not dissolve in water but is partly broken down by fermentation. Crucially, it is the main food source of gut microbes, and it helps keep things moving along the digestive tract, helping avoid digestive problems. It is found in foods including whole grains and vegetables. The fermentation of undigested fiber (both soluble and insoluble) in the gut creates short-chain fatty acids, which have many health benefits (see p.69).

Cellulose bond structure

Cellulose is the most abundant carbohydrate present in nature and is indigestible. Chains of glucose monomers are connected by glycidic bonds, which can't be broken down.

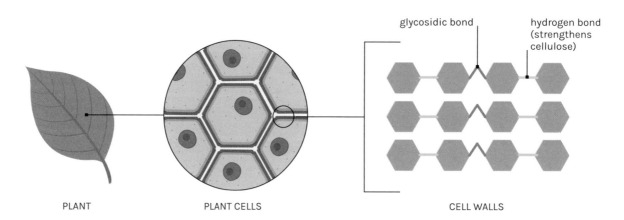

glycosidic bond

hydrogen bond (strengthens cellulose)

PLANT   PLANT CELLS   CELL WALLS

Fiber-rich vegetables
Eating a diverse range of fruits and vegetables will help you reach the recommended 30g of fiber a day.

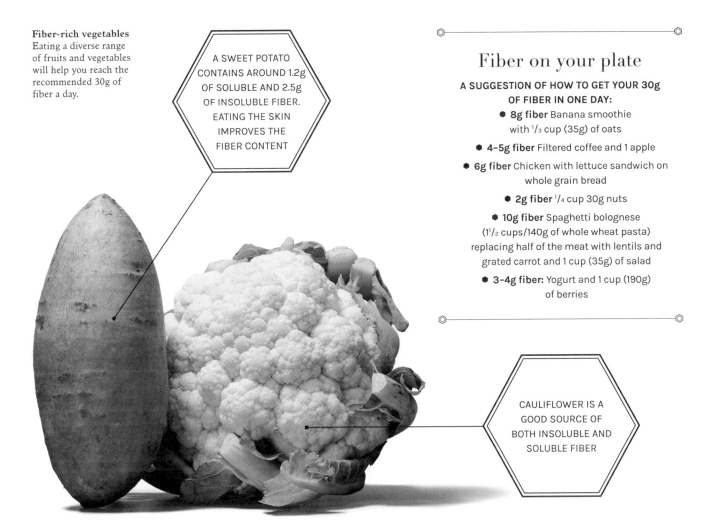

A SWEET POTATO CONTAINS AROUND 1.2g OF SOLUBLE AND 2.5g OF INSOLUBLE FIBER. EATING THE SKIN IMPROVES THE FIBER CONTENT

Fiber on your plate

A SUGGESTION OF HOW TO GET YOUR 30g OF FIBER IN ONE DAY:

- **8g fiber** Banana smoothie with ¹/₃ cup (35g) of oats
- **4–5g fiber** Filtered coffee and 1 apple
- **6g fiber** Chicken with lettuce sandwich on whole grain bread
- **2g fiber** ¹/₄ cup 30g nuts
- **10g fiber** Spaghetti bolognese (1¹/₂ cups/140g of whole wheat pasta) replacing half of the meat with lentils and grated carrot and 1 cup (35g) of salad
- **3–4g fiber:** Yogurt and 1 cup (190g) of berries

CAULIFLOWER IS A GOOD SOURCE OF BOTH INSOLUBLE AND SOLUBLE FIBER

FIBER FACTS

The recommendation is that adults eat around 30g of fiber in their diet every day. Younger children should aim for 15–20g a day and teenagers around 25g a day. If more people consumed a whole plant-food diet, the numbers reaching the target of 30g a day would improve drastically. A study of over 400,000 participants found that those with the higher intake of whole grains had a 20 percent reduced risk of heart disease compared with those who had a lower fiber intake. An increase of 8g more fiber a day can reduce our risk of colon cancer by 8 percent, risk of type 2 diabetes by 15 percent, risk of heart disease by 19 percent, and overall risk of death by 7 percent. Furthermore, for every 15g increase of whole grains eaten per day, total deaths and incidences of coronary heart disease, type 2 diabetes, and colorectal cancer decrease by up to 19 percent. Although 30g a day may be the target, exceeding that could provide us all with even better protection for our health.

If increasing the fiber in your diet, add it slowly and drink plenty of water because a sudden increase can cause problems such as bloating and loose bowel movements. You may want to seek the supervision of a doctor or nutritionist before making such a change.

WHAT ARE THE BENEFITS OF PREBIOTIC AND PROBIOTIC FOODS?

Although humans have eaten prebiotic and probiotic foods for thousands of years as part of their everyday diet, we are only just realizing the health benefits they can deliver. But what are they, and how can they help us?

———————

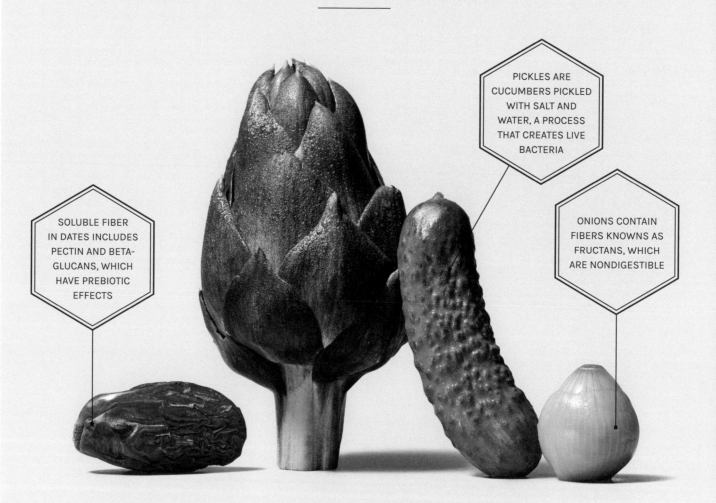

PICKLES ARE CUCUMBERS PICKLED WITH SALT AND WATER, A PROCESS THAT CREATES LIVE BACTERIA

ONIONS CONTAIN FIBERS KNOWNS AS FRUCTANS, WHICH ARE NONDIGESTIBLE

SOLUBLE FIBER IN DATES INCLUDES PECTIN AND BETA-GLUCANS, WHICH HAVE PREBIOTIC EFFECTS

THE 4 Ks

One way to remember some of the most popular groups of probiotic foods is to think of the four Ks. Adding some or all of these to your diet will support your gut microbiota.

WHAT ARE PREBIOTICS?

Prebiotics are a type of fiber you get from food that help healthy bacteria grow in your gut. It is worth noting that not all fibers are prebiotics. Prebiotic fibers are resistant to the acidic conditions of the stomach and remain undigested until they reach the colon. They are then fermented by the intestinal microbiota and are able to change the growth or activity of the microbiota. Examples of prebiotic foods are:

- Fruits, including apples, dates, prunes, dried mango, pears, grapefruit, and apricots
- Vegetables such as onions, leeks, garlic, pulses, beans, both Jerusalem and globe artichokes (pictured, right), chicory root, and asparagus
- Other foods like wheat bran, cashews, pistachios, black tea, chai, and fennel tea.

WHAT ARE PROBIOTICS?

Probiotics are live strains of bacteria found in fermented foods that can be consumed to directly increase the population of "good" bacteria in the gut. Examples of probiotics are yogurts, miso, kefir, kombuch, kimchi, and sauerkraut. If buying yogurts or probiotic drinks, check the label to make sure they contain specific "friendly" bacterial strains, often from the *Lactobacillus* and *Bifidobacteria* species. Good-quality cheese also contains some probiotic bacteria if it is made using fermented milk. Synbiotics are supplements that contain both prebiotics and probiotics.

POPULAR PROBIOTIC FOODS

In recent years, probiotic supplements have risen in popularity, and you can buy many supplements and drinks claiming a range of benefits. However, many of these are not regulated so it is safer and less expensive to consume probiotics through food, such as yogurt. Some probiotics, such as sauerkraut and kefir, can be made fairy easily at home.

WHAT ARE THE BENEFITS?

Probiotics appear to have many benefits both for our gut health and overall health. They may help improve symptoms of irritable bowel syndrome (IBS) as well as help prevent life-threatening diseases, such as necrotizing enterocolitis (a serious illness in which tissues in the intestine become inflamed and start to die) in premature infants. There is evidence that consuming probiotics while using antibiotics reduces the risk of antibiotic-related diarrhea by 60 percent. There may also be a link between probiotics and improved mental health, including depression; a reduction in respiratory illnesses such as ventilator-associated pneumonia; eczema flares; vaginal infections; and gestational diabetes.

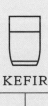

KEFIR

A drink made from fermented milk. Contains both prebiotics and probiotics. Vegan versions are available.

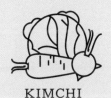

KIMCHI

A classic Korean side dish of fermented vegetables, such as cabbage, radishes, and carrots, flavored with red chile pepper flakes.

KOMBUCHA

A fermented drink made with black or green tea, sugar, bacteria, and yeast. Often carbonated with a slightly sour taste.

KRAUT

Finely cut raw cabbage with salt added, which causes a fermentation process using naturally present lactic acid bacteria.

SHOULD WE EAT FERMENTED FOODS?

Fermented foods have grown in popularity in recent years. They are known to be beneficial, in particular for gut health, by supporting our gut microbiota. What are fermented foods, and why should we eat them?

WHAT IS FERMENTATION?

Fermentation is a natural process by which sugar in food is changed into alcohol, organic acids, or gases by bacteria, yeast, or fungi. Throughout history, it has been used as a way of preserving and making products, including beer and bread. Around 35 percent of our diets today depend upon foods that have been fermented, such as chocolate, coffee, cheese, alcohol, and bread. However, not all fermented foods benefit the gut bacteria as they don't contain living microbes due to the processes they undergo (such as the cooking process used when baking bread).

WHAT ARE THE BENEFITS?

Many health benefits are linked to the consumption of fermented foods. Importantly, they could increase the diversity of beneficial bacteria strains in the gut and break down food into short-chain fatty acids including butyrate, acetate, and propionate (see p.69), which are good for our overall health. The consumption of lactic acid bacteria via fermented foods may also help modulate the gut microbiome and its stress response. Fermented foods such as sauerkraut and kimchi contain fiber, which promotes the growth of beneficial bacteria in the gut. Kefir, kombucha, and tempeh all produce anti-inflammatory compounds during fermentation, which are beneficial to health.

Fermented foods also contain beneficial organic acids that impact blood pressure and may potentially help with blood sugar control. Studies have shown that IBS symptoms have been helped by the daily consumption of 3oz (75g) of sauerkraut, but more research is needed. Another area of nutritional research has shown that some molecules found in

---

Fermented foods

Apart from the four Ks (see pp.76–77), there are many more unusual fermented foods available that you can seek out to add variety to your diet and increase the diversity of bacteria in your gut.

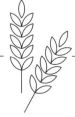

NURUNGJI

A Korean dish made by crisping the layer of scorched rice at the bottom of a pot, then rehydrating it with water.

KVASS

A fermented drink made from bread that contains a low amount of alcohol. Popular in Russia.

NATTO

Made from soybeans fermented with *Bacillus subtilis*. Popular in Japanese cuisine.

Lactic acid and alcoholic fermentation

Lactic acid fermentation is a process by which sugars are converted into lactic acid and is used in the production of fermented food. In alcoholic fermentation, glucose creates an airy structure in and imparts flavor to bread and other products by the yeast *Saccharomyces*.

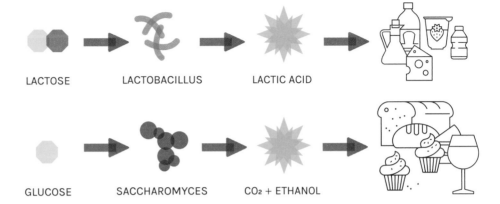

LACTOSE → LACTOBACILLUS → LACTIC ACID →

GLUCOSE → SACCHAROMYCES → CO₂ + ETHANOL →

fermented foods, for instance gamma-aminobutyric acids (GABA), are known to have a relaxing impact on the brain so may help improve mental health. There may be benefits for those with intolerances to gluten and lactose because the fermentation process can lower the content of those proteins and sugars in some sourdough breads. Some aged cheeses, such as Cheddar, Swiss, and Parmesan, are also typically low in lactose due to fermentation.

Remember, as with any change in diet, make changes slowly and increase your intake of water to prevent digestive discomfort.

A note of caution

STORE-BOUGHT VERSUS HOMEMADE.
It is important to be aware of the limitations of some claims made about fermented food and drink. The benefits from commercially fermented food may be minimal as you cannot be sure of the processes used. If you do buy store-bought, check that the product is unpasteurized so that you can be sure it contains live microbes. A potent homemade version of fermented foods is likely to be better than the type you buy in the supermarket. Check the internet for ideas on making your own pickles or sauerkraut.

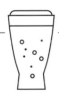

CIDER

Yeast transforms the sucrose, fructose, and glucose of the apples into the alcohol.

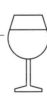

WINE

Through the process of fermentation, grape juice is turned into an alcoholic beverage.

MISO

A thick paste made by fermenting soybeans with salt and koji (a type of fungus).

BAMBOO SHOOTS

Used in Asian cooking, fermented bamboo shoots are added to pickles and salads for flavor.

CAN YOU HAVE TOO MUCH FIBER?

Currently most people are not getting enough fiber in their diets in western countries let alone having too much. There are many benefits to adding fiber to your meals and it is unlikely that you will consume too much of it.

Fiber can be described by its physical characteristics such as how thick it is, how well it dissolves, and how well it breaks down inside the body—known as fermentability. The two main types are soluble and insoluble fiber (see pp.74–75).

FIBER INTAKE

Fiber is without doubt important for our health, but most of us in the Western world do not consume enough of it, so it is unlikely that you're eating too much of it. Globally, it is generally recommended that we consume 20–30g of fiber a day from food.

The average intake in the US is around 15g a day in adults, but it is not harmful to exceed that amount if your body has adapted to it.

It is believed that our ancestors might have consumed up to 150g of fiber a day, although this may have been due to a limited choice of food available rather than out of choice. Studies of the present-day Hadza hunter-gatherer tribes in Tanzania, who eat a diet higher in fiber than most people today, have shown that they have a more diverse gut microbiome than their industrialized countries' urban-dwelling counterparts.

Fiber-rich plant foods

Try to include as many of these foods as possible in your diet on a regular basis to make sure that you're eating enough fiber. Many of these are also good sources of protein (see pp.94–95).

Bulgur wheat
A whole grain wheat with a nutty flavor and chewy texture.

Chickpeas
Also known as garbanzo beans, can be used to make hummus.

Green peas
A legume that is rich in nutrients and protein. Good fresh or frozen.

Oats
A whole grain high in soluble fiber, especially beta glucans which is good for heart health.

Adzuki beans
Versatile, small red-brown beans with a nutty flavor used in many Asian dishes.

White beans
Such as cannellini and butter beans. Use in soups, stews, and pasta dishes.

Red kidney beans
Contain iron, potassium, and protein. Use canned or dried in chilies and with rice.

Broccoli
Versatile and rich in vitamins and minerals. Try steamed, boiled, stir-fried, or raw.

ADD FIBER GRADUALLY

If you are changing your diet and adding more fiber, this may result in gastric distress, often manifesting itself as excess gas and bloating. Some foods such as Jerusalem artichokes contain a prebiotic called inulin, which can cause flatulence and diarrhea. To avoid this, increase fiber gradually rather than all at once. At the same time, boost your water consumption to help you remain hydrated—too much fiber without water can result in dehydration and uncomfortable hard stools as water helps soften them.

WILL FIBER CAUSE BLOATING?

Eating high-fiber foods, such as pulses, may lead to bloating as there is more gas production in the large intestine, although fiber can also reduce bloating as it helps improve digestion and moves food more quickly through the gut. If you're suffering from bloating, this may be caused by excess fiber and a number of other issues, including stress, hormones, constipation, sensitive gut, and IBS

Causes of bloating

There are many causes of bloating, and it is a very common condition. Eating the right amount of fiber will not usually cause bloating, as long as you increase your intake gradually and drink plenty of water.

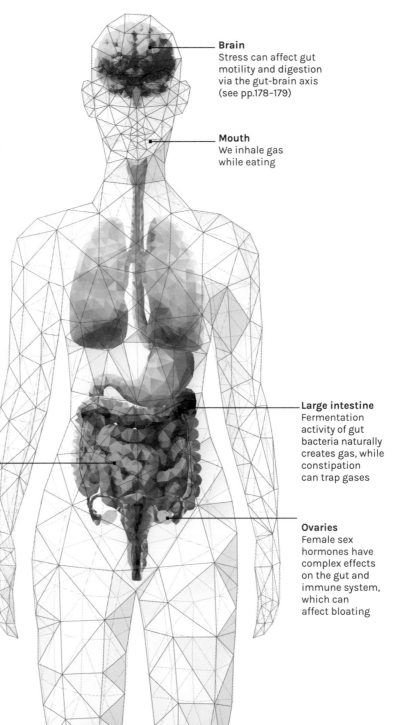

Brain
Stress can affect gut motility and digestion via the gut-brain axis (see pp.178–179)

Mouth
We inhale gas while eating

Large intestine
Fermentation activity of gut bacteria naturally creates gas, while constipation can trap gases

Ovaries
Female sex hormones have complex effects on the gut and immune system, which can affect bloating

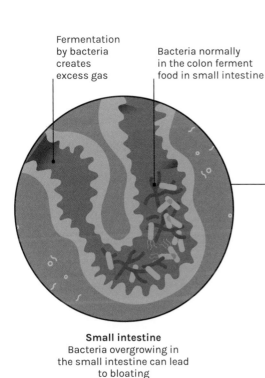

Fermentation by bacteria creates excess gas

Bacteria normally in the colon ferment food in small intestine

Small intestine
Bacteria overgrowing in the small intestine can lead to bloating

IS A PLANT-BASED DIET GOOD FOR IBS?

Globally, 5–10 percent of people suffer from some sort of digestive discomfort or irritable bowel syndrome (IBS). Diet is the most important strategy for dealing with these issues, but does eating a plant-based diet help IBS or make it worse?

WHAT IS IBS?

Irritable bowel syndrome, or IBS, is a condition where people suffer a range of issues, including bloating, constipation, and/or diarrhea, and recurrent pain in the abdomen. It can be a difficult condition to diagnose, and patients must have suffered frequent abdominal pain for at least three months, with some further symptoms for at least six months, before diagnosis. There is no specific test to diagnose IBS; it's often a case of ruling out digestive diseases first with your doctor and then concluding that it is IBS. There are certain factors that can increase your risk of getting IBS, such as having a recent gut infection, "travelers' diarrhea," and food poisoning.

HOW IBS IS MANAGED

IBS can be improved by looking at how and what you eat in order to support the gut, keeping a food diary, identifying triggers, and reducing common causes such as spicy foods, caffeine, alcohol, deep-fried foods high in fat, and artificial sweeteners. The advice is to reduce fiber intake from fruits and vegetables and to consume it across the day, slowly building the amount. For 50 percent of those with IBS, this approach is often effective, but others may need more help.

THE FODMAP APPROACH

FODMAPs are a group of indigestible carbohydrates fermented in the large intestine: fermentable, oligosaccharides,

Stomach

Small intestine

Large intestine

FODMAPs in the gut

FODMAPs may trigger excess water to be drawn into the large intestine, and ferment, producing gas, causing discomfort and other symptoms.

FOODS HIGH IN FODMAPS

Garlic, onions, mushrooms, apples, pears, watermelon, cherries, and wheat products such as pasta and pastries are all classed as FODMAP foods disaccharides, monosaccharides, and polyols. These carbohydrates are not absorbed well by our small intestine, which can end up in the large intestine, causing excess fluid and fermentation-causing gas. The low-FODMAP diet (LFD) is a way of controlling the amount of these foods consumed and includes plant foods such as kale, tofu, and tempeh. Following a low-FODMAP diet is a complex three-stage process and must be supervised by a trained health professional. First, you eliminate or restrict all FODMAPs from the diet; second, you reintroduce one or two foods at a time and see what effect this has. Finally, you personalize your diet, adding back FODMAPs that don't have an adverse effect.

PLANT-BASED IBS DIETS

Eating a plant-based diet brings many health benefits, although it is not clear whether it has any positive benefits for IBS sufferers in particular. However, if you are able to tolerate a slow increase in plant-based foods in your diet, it will mean a promotion of good bacteria in your gut. Understanding which plants work well for you, eating a variety of foods, cooking in a certain way, and adopting movement and lifestyle strategies can be helpful for your gut microbes. Following a plant-based diet and the low-FODMAP diet at the same time may lead to social restrictions and nutritional deficiencies but can be done safely with the right support and advice from a dietitian.

Low-FODMAP alternatives

YOU CAN ADAPT THE LOW-FODMAP DIET TO SUIT A PLANT-BASED DIET.
A FODMAP "gentle" approach may be easier and lead to fewer restrictions for those following a plant-based diet—this involves removing a few very high FODMAP foods rather than following the full diet that excludes all high FODMAP foods. The best way is usually to increase your intake of plant foods slowly and monitor the effect they have on you.

FODMAPs

LOW-FODMAP FOODS INCLUDE QUINOA, BROCCOLI, SPINACH, OATS, NUTS, EDAMAME, PUMPKIN SEEDS

F
FERMENTABLE

O
OLIGOSACCHARIDES

D
DISACCHARIDES

M
MONOSACCHARIDES

A
AND

P
POLYOLS

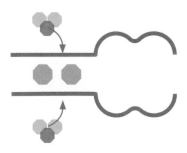

SMALL INTESTINE

FODMAPs cause water to be drawn into the large intestine, leading to distension and bloating

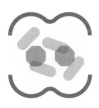

BACTERIAL REACTION IN LARGE INTESTINE

Bacteria in the large intestine ferment FODMAPs, which leads to gas production

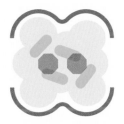

GAS BUILDS UP = EXPANSION

The muscle wall expands with the buildup of gas as a result of the fermentation

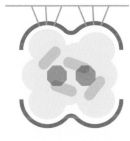

MESSAGE SENT TO NERVOUS SYSTEM

The large intestine sends a signal via the expanded muscle to the nervous system, causing pain

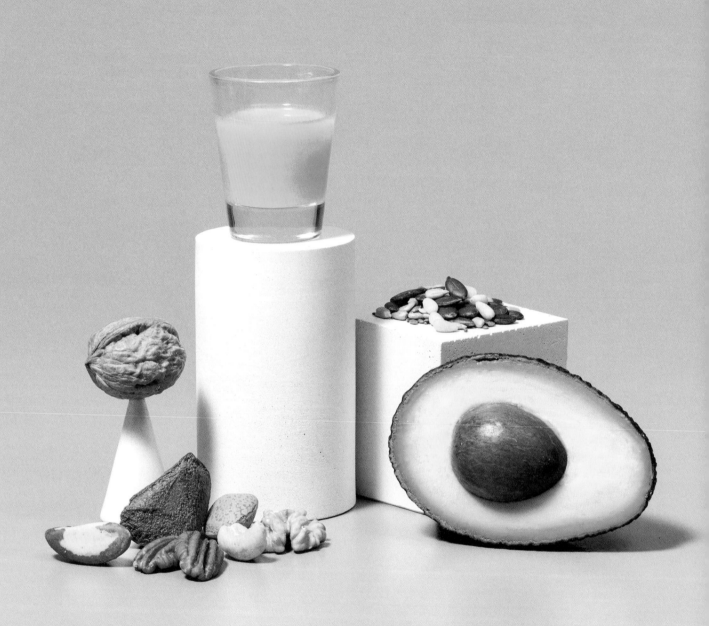

OBTAINING NUTRIENTS

WHY ARE NUTRIENTS SO IMPORTANT FOR HEALTH?

In order to maintain optimum health, we need to consume the correct nutrients to supply our body with the energy and components it needs to function well. How much of each nutrient we need depends on different factors.

WHAT ARE NUTRIENTS?

The World Health Organization states that a nutrient is a substance we need to aid the body's survival, growth, and reproduction. These processes are carried out by chemical compounds created in the body, but your body cannot create all of the compounds it needs without essential nutrients. You require a lot of nutrition to enable your body to work tirelessly every day performing many functions simultaneously.

All food contains nutrients in the form of macronutrients and micronutrients. The macronutrients are fats, protein, and carbohydrates (see pp.20–21), and the micronutrients are vitamins and minerals (see pp.22–23). We need a combination of these nutrients and water on a daily basis to be as healthy as possible. As the name suggests, you need to eat larger amounts of macronutrients on a daily basis. Micronutrients are needed in smaller amounts but are vital in order to maintain a healthy body.

NUTRIENT REQUIREMENTS

Everyone has different needs when it comes to nutrients. Much of this depends on your age and gender as well as your levels of physical activity, your general health and well-being, your dietary habits, as well as your genetic makeup. For example, as women go through menstruation and menopause, their requirements change and they need more iron and unsaturated fatty acids. People who are more active need more calories than those who live a more sedentary lifestyle. Also, those with a lactose intolerance or who are vegan may need to get the vitamins and minerals usually found in dairy from other sources.

Daily amounts

Recommended Dietary Intake (RDI) is the average daily intake of a particular nutrient that should meet the nutritional requirements of 97–98 percent of healthy adults.

RDIs are based on gender and age. Reference intakes aren't meant to be targets but can be a useful way of showing how products could fit into a diet. On food labels, they show what percentage contribution a particular product or portion size of your daily reference intake the food contains. In this way, it can help to encourage healthier eating. There are no recommended dietary intakes for children.

NUTRIENT DEFICIENCIES

Avoiding deficiencies is key to supporting our immune system and enabling us to be free from disease. The body's immune response relies on the presence of many micronutrients. Some vitamins and minerals that have been identified as crucial for the growth and function of immune cells include vitamin C, vitamin D, zinc, selenium (see pp.22–23), iron (see pp.98–99), and protein (including the amino acid glutamine; see pp.92–93). The recommended intake of key nutrients laid out by public health guidelines in various countries represents the minimum intake of the nutrient to be well, healthy, and free from poor health.

What nutrients do for us

The nutrients we consume through food help us stay alive They are used as an energy source, to heal, build, and repair tissue. Nutrients also sustain growth, help transport oxygen to cells, and regulate bodily functions.

BRAIN FUNCTION

Nutrients are critical for proper brain function, memory, and cognitive processes. Essential fatty acids, vitamins, and minerals, such as omega-3 fatty acids and B vitamins, are important for brain health.

ENERGY PRODUCTION

Nutrients, especially macronutrients like carbohydrates, proteins, and fats, provide the energy needed for daily activities, metabolic processes, and overall vitality.

GROWTH AND DEVELOPMENT

Nutrients, particularly during childhood and adolescence, support growth, tissue repair, and the development of various body structures.

CELLULAR FUNCTION

Nutrients are essential for the proper functioning of cells, including cellular communication, transport of molecules, and the production of energy (in the form of adenosine triphosphate or ATP).

DIGESTION

Nutrients are needed for the proper functioning of the digestive system, including the breakdown of food and absorption of nutrients from the gastrointestinal tract.

IMMUNE FUNCTION

Many nutrients, such as vitamins and minerals, are important for a strong immune system. They help the body fight off infections and diseases.

REPAIR AND MAINTENANCE

Nutrients are required for the repair and maintenance of tissues, especially during times of injury or illness.

METABOLISM

Nutrients are involved in metabolic processes such as the breakdown of food, absorption of nutrients, and the regulation of hormones and enzymes.

BONE HEALTH

Nutrients like calcium, vitamin D, and vitamin K are crucial for maintaining strong and healthy bones.

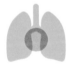

HEALTHY TISSUES AND ORGANS

Nutrients play a role in maintaining the health of various tissues and organs, including the skin, eyes, bones, and organs like the heart and liver.

HORMONE PRODUCTION

Several nutrients, such as vitamins and minerals, are involved in the production and regulation of hormones that control various bodily functions.

DETOXIFICATION

Some nutrients are involved in the body's natural detoxification processes, helping remove waste and toxins from the body.

WHAT AFFECTS NUTRIENT BIOAVAILABILITY?

In order to get the most out of what we eat, we need to ensure we are effectively absorbing the food we eat. The amount of a nutrient that is absorbed and used by the body is called bioavailability. This often means pairing up food to help this process and looking after our bodies' needs.

When we eat, we don't simply take all of the nutrition from the food we consume; our bodies take what they need and excrete the remainder with a highly efficient detoxification system. Nutrient absorption is quite complex; the assimilation of substances like vitamins, minerals, fatty acids, and amino acids into the bloodstream and cells or across tissue and organs takes a lot of work. This involves many types of enzymes, saliva, acid, bile, and more (see pp.12–13). Most nutrients from food and supplements pass through the wall of the small intestine and into the blood vessels where they are carried elsewhere as needed.

MALABSORPTION

Sometimes nutrients are not absorbed well and require other nutrients to work with them to aid this process, or our bodies don't work as efficiently as they should. When the ability to absorb some or all nutrients (carbs, proteins, fats, vitamins, and minerals) is impaired, this is known as malabsorption, and it can impact our digestive system and cause varying degrees of distress. Over the course of our lives, we are all likely to experience issues relating to our digestive system. Digestive concerns such as bloating, gas, nausea, vomiting, and diarrhea are common. In the short term, malabsorption will cause gastrointestinal distress; over time, your body will start to show signs of deficiency in unabsorbed nutrients. It is important you speak to your primary care provider if you are concerned as deficiencies in macronutrients will lead to undernutrition, which can be seen through muscle wasting, reduced immunity, unintentional weight

Nutrient absorption

The process of nutrient absorption begins as soon as you take food into your mouth and begin chewing. As it moves through the digestive system, our enzymes get to work to break down the food into carbs, proteins, fats, vitamins, and minerals, which can be used to fuel your metabolism.

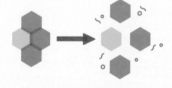

INGESTION

As you chew your food, it breaks into smaller pieces, and enzymes in the saliva start breaking it down before you swallow.

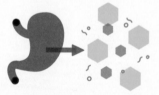

STOMACH

When the food reaches your stomach, it is further broken down into chyme by the enzymes in the gastric juices.

loss, and anemia. Deficiencies of micronutrients may affect your bones, skin, hair, and eye health. Factors that affect nutrient absorption include:

- The natural aging process
- Food intolerances, such as gluten or lactose intolerance, for example (see pp.198–199)
- Eating an inflammatory diet that contains high levels of processed foods, sugar, and fat
- Chronic stress
- Dehydration/overhydration
- Eating quickly
- Tannins—these are found in beans, lentils, greens, tea, and coffee. Some research suggests that these components reduce iron absorption, but the benefits of consuming them (for their antioxidant and anti-inflammatory properties) outweigh this problem. Avoid drinking tea or coffee to avoid malabsorption.

WHAT CAN I DO TO AID ABSORPTION?

To maximize nutrient intake, try the following:

- Consume probiotics, (see pp.76–77), which may be beneficial in supporting our gut microbiota to support digestion.

- Ensure you are eating mindfully and fully chewing food, as this helps digestive enzymes release, which is key to digestion.
- Manage stress levels—this is easier said than done, but stress actively alters hormones, which can draw blood flow away from the digestive process, impacting hunger and fullness signals.
- Stay hydrated. We need water to help the small intestine with a process known as diffusion. This process moves water-soluble compounds, such as glucose, amino acids, and micronutrients, including vitamins B and C, across barriers like the villi. These nutrients then enter the bloodstream, where they can be used as energy (with the exception of fat-soluble vitamins A, D, E, and K, which need a few extra steps before entering the bloodstream).

There is also some data to suggest calcium supplementation can decrease iron absorption short term, but again this isn't a reason to stop taking this important supplement if required. By increasing vitamin C, you should be able to increase the uptake of iron (see pp.100–101).

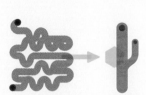

SMALL INTESTINE

Most of the nutrients are absorbed from the small intestine through the villi and into the bloodstream.

LARGE INTESTINE

In the large intestine, water is absorbed, and any indigestible matter is formed into feces.

ELIMINATION

Any waste that remains is removed from the body through the rectum and anus.

HOW CAN I MAXIMIZE NUTRIENT BIOAVAILABILITY?

There are a few simple things we can do to aid nutrient absorption, including the way we eat, what we eat, and how we pair foods together to maximize our nutrition. The way our food is prepared also plays a role in nutrient absorption.

———

Planning your diet well and eating a lot of whole foods with balanced plates will support nutrient absorption. Knowing which foods work well together will help you maximize the nutrients you consume.

INTERACTION OF NUTRIENTS IN THE BODY

Some nutrients are better absorbed in tandem with others. Here are some examples of those that work well together for effective absorption:

• **Iron and vitamin C** Some dietary factors have been shown to enhance the absorption of iron from foods, such as ascorbic acid (also known as vitamin C). It's not enough to eat a daily diet that contains both nutrients—absorption of the iron will be much greater if the nutrients are paired in a single meal, according to research published in the *American Journal of Clinical Nutrition*.

• **Calcium and vitamin D** We need vitamin D to help calcium enter our bloodstream and kidneys, and for our gut to absorb it. Therefore, if we are deficient in vitamin D, we are also likely deficient in calcium (see pp. 104–105). Having adequate amounts of vitamin D, equol (soy), monounsaturated fats, fiber, inulin (a soluble fiber found in Jerusalem artichokes and chicory root), phosphorus, iron, and magnesium has been linked to increasing calcium absorption, as have dairy foods fortified with calcium.

• **Turmeric and black pepper** The key compounds in turmeric are called curcuminoids. Curcumin itself

Food preparation

How we prepare food may affect how well we are able to absorb the nutrients it contains. Some of the key methods of preparing foods to aid bioavailability are shown here.

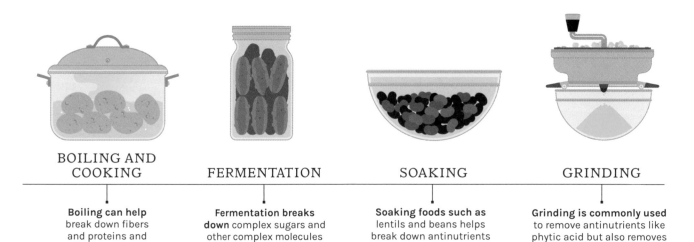

BOILING AND COOKING
Boiling can help break down fibers and proteins and release enzymes.

FERMENTATION
Fermentation breaks down complex sugars and other complex molecules into simpler forms.

SOAKING
Soaking foods such as lentils and beans helps break down antinutrients and aids digestion.

GRINDING
Grinding is commonly used to remove antinutrients like phytic acid but also removes other nutrients.

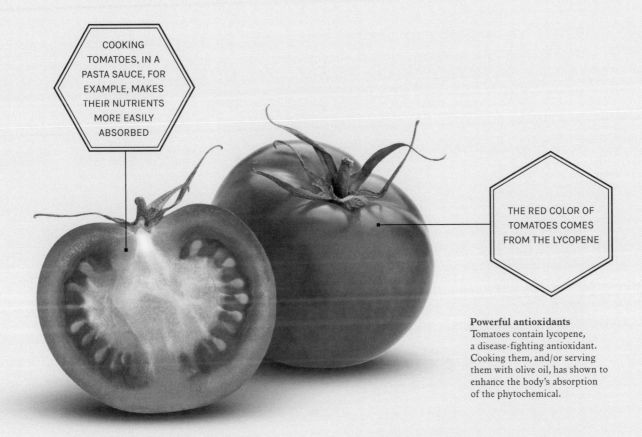

COOKING TOMATOES, IN A PASTA SAUCE, FOR EXAMPLE, MAKES THEIR NUTRIENTS MORE EASILY ABSORBED

THE RED COLOR OF TOMATOES COMES FROM THE LYCOPENE

Powerful antioxidants
Tomatoes contain lycopene, a disease-fighting antioxidant. Cooking them, and/or serving them with olive oil, has shown to enhance the body's absorption of the phytochemical.

is the most active ingredient and appears to be the most important, but it is not easily absorbed by the body. One study showed that adding 20mg of piperine (found in black pepper) to 2g of curcumin increased its absorption significantly.

- **Vitamins and fat** Some vitamins (such as vitamins A, D, E, and K) are fat-soluble and require fat to be effectively absorbed in our intestines. For example, to increase absorption of vitamin A from sweet potatoes, pair them with butter or avocado. Getting enough of these vitamins and maximally absorbing them is important because deficiencies are connected with heightened risk of cancer and type 2 diabetes.

ANTINUTRIENTS

Some plant foods contain antinutrients, which reduce the absorption of nutrients into the bloodstream. These include phytic acids (phytates), tannins, protease inhibitors, and lectins. By cooking and preparing food in different ways, we can reduce the effect of antinutrients (see pp.152–153).

GROWING OLDER

As we age, key nutrients can become harder to absorb. Reasons for this include changes to the digestive system, reduced appetite, changes to taste and smell, and the use of medication. One study of the elderly suggested including more of the following could help improve nutrient density:

- **Vitamin A:** Carrots, leeks, pumpkins
- **Vitamin B1:** Peas and bananas
- **Vitamin B2:** Mushrooms and eggs
- **Vitamin B6:** Chickpeas, avocado, and sweet potato
- **Vitamin B12 and calcium:** Add skim milk powder to foods
- **Zinc:** Lentils, chickpeas, seeds, and whole grains
- **Selenium:** Nuts, eggs, or fish-based dishes.

WILL I STRUGGLE TO EAT ENOUGH PROTEIN?

Many people worry that if they don't eat meat, their diet will lack protein.
However, if a plant-based diet is considered and planned well,
it is entirely possible to get enough protein.

A lot of research has been done on vegetarian diets that suggests appropriately planned plant-based diets can easily provide all of our protein needs.

HOW MUCH PROTEIN DO I NEED?

The recommendation for protein for adult male vegans is around 63g per day; for adult female vegans, it is around 52g per day, and this is surprisingly easy to obtain if you're eating a balanced diet.

Plant sources of protein include beans, peas, lentils, nuts, seeds, whole grains, and soy foods. Meat substitutes like vegetarian burgers, soy sausages, and other meat alternatives can be useful for those adapting to a plant-based diet and can provide a source of protein (see pp. 60–61). However, as with any processed foods, these can often be high in salt and fat so should be used in moderation. These products may also contain animal ingredients such as eggs, milk derivatives, and honey, so read labels carefully if you wish to follow a vegan diet.

PLANT-BASED PROTEINS

Some plant-based foods contain all the essential amino acids, such as those in the following list:

- soy foods (tofu or tempeh, for example)
- quinoa
- hemp seeds
- chia seeds
- mycoprotein/Quorn

The amino acid content varies in other plant-based foods and you won't always get a complete profile, but as long as your diet is diverse and you consume a range of protein sources, your body will pull together what it needs. The foods listed opposite are just a few examples of the kinds of foods you could include in your diet.

Top 10 protein sources from plant foods

Try to include these foods in your diet to ensure that you're getting enough amino acids, the building blocks of protein. The protein values are per 100g.

SEITAN

A good source of plant protein made from wheat gluten.

27–75g PROTEIN

TOFU

Made from curdled soy milk.

8–15g PROTEIN

TEMPEH

Made from fermented soybeans.

18–21g PROTEIN

QUORN

A complete protein source derived from fungus that is low in fat.

10–20g PROTEIN

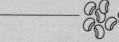

KIDNEY BEANS

Rich in protein and high in fiber, a great addition to chili and salads.

8–9g PROTEIN

The nine essential amino acids

These are the essential amino acids that your body needs to function. You don't need to eat foods with amino acids at every meal, but you need to get a balance of them through a varied diet on a regular basis.

HISTIDINE
is used for creation of blood cells, growth, and tissue repair. It is found in sunflower and pumpkin seeds, rice, chickpeas, and lentils.

ISOLEUCINE
is vital for immune function, muscle metabolism, and energy regulation. You can get it from kidney beans, lentils, and chickpeas.

LEUCINE
is a regulator of muscle protein synthesis needed for wound healing, regulating blood sugar levels, and growth. Found in soybeans.

TRYPTOPHAN
is important for the production of serotonin. It can be found in sesame, pumpkin, and sunflower seeds.

LYSINE
helps produce enzymes, antibodies, and hormones. It also helps with collagen formation and calcium absorption. It is found in pistachio nuts.

THREONINE
plays an important role in maintaining your skin and teeth. You can find this in haricot beans and sweet potatoes.

METHIONINE
helps the body's detoxification and metabolism. You can get it from almonds and Brazil nuts.

PHENYLALANINE
helps create other amino acids such as tyrosine, used in the production of dopamine. Found in spinach and bananas.

VALINE
is involved in energy production and helps support the nervous system. It is found in chickpeas, almonds, and peanuts.

CHICKPEAS

Rich in protein and can be used in a variety of plant-based dishes.

8g PROTEIN

WHOLE GRAIN PASTA

Helps boost protein intake.

4g PROTEIN

ALMONDS

Almonds are one of the highest protein nuts alongside pistachios.

21g PROTEIN

HEMP SEEDS

Add to smoothies, salads, and yogurts to boost protein.

31g PROTEIN

QUINOA

A nutrient-packed pseudograin, useful in salads.

4g PROTEIN

WILL I CONSUME TOO MANY CARBOHYDRATES?

It is possible to consume too many carbs whether you are eating a plant-based diet or not. Carbohydrates have been demonized over the years, with many choosing to eat a low-carb diet to lose weight, but they are an essential part of our diet, providing the body with energy in the form of glucose.

ARE CARBS BAD FOR YOU?

Carbohydrates are not bad for us; they are a vital source of energy and are an important part of our diet for optimum health and well-being (see pp.20–21), but the quantity and quality of the carbohydrates you eat dictates the overall health outcome. Avoid eating carbs that don't contain fiber, and watch for added sugar. Examples of these are white bread, white pasta, white rice, breakfast cereals, and chips. It is easy to eat too many of these refined carbs because they contain added sugar and fat, which is very appealing to the taste buds. If the carbohydrates you consume are mainly from ultra-processed foods, you are also consuming salt, sugar, and fat, which is detrimental to long-term health for a variety of reasons (see pp.30–31).

HOW MUCH SHOULD I EAT?

In the US, it is recommended that you get between 45 to 65 percent of your overall calories from carbohydrates—this equates to roughly 225–325g per day on the generic 2,000 calorie a day diet.

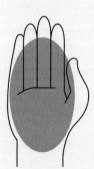

3–4
SERVINGS OF STARCHY CARBOHYDRATES

1 SERVING

= 2 handfuls dried rice/pasta/couscous (less for 4 servings)

= 1 fist-size baked potato

= 2 slices bread

Serving sizes have increased dramatically over the past 40 years. As a general rule, a serving about the size of your fist is an appropriate mealtime portion of carbohydrate-containing foods, and you should aim for 3–4 servings per day. This can then be adjusted depending on your activity levels. It is recommended that starchy foods should make up just over a third of the food you eat. However, this varies depending on your body size, age, and other factors. We don't all need to consume 2,000 calories a day; some people may need more or fewer calories. There may be a variety of advisable carbohydrate ranges based upon your unique activity levels, needs, and requirements.

CHOOSING THE RIGHT CARBS

If you include whole food carbohydrates in your daily diet that contain fiber, vitamins, minerals, and phytonutrients, it is less likely that you will overconsume carbs. This will also keep a check on your blood sugar levels and avoid major glucose spikes (see pp.172–173). Some whole food carbs to look out for include:

- Vegetables
- Legumes
- Whole grains
- Fruit

You can make informed choices that will reduce your overall carbohydrate intake if you are trying to lose weight. However, it is best to still eat a variety of foods and a balanced diet instead of cutting out carbs altogether.

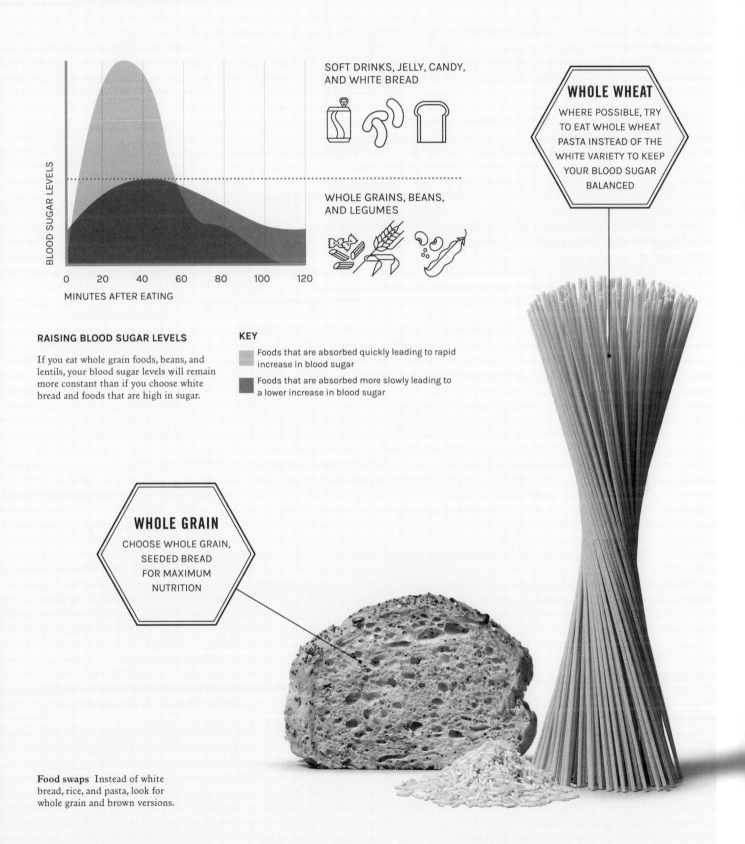

BLOOD SUGAR LEVELS

MINUTES AFTER EATING

SOFT DRINKS, JELLY, CANDY, AND WHITE BREAD

WHOLE GRAINS, BEANS, AND LEGUMES

RAISING BLOOD SUGAR LEVELS

If you eat whole grain foods, beans, and lentils, your blood sugar levels will remain more constant than if you choose white bread and foods that are high in sugar.

KEY

Foods that are absorbed quickly leading to rapid increase in blood sugar

Foods that are absorbed more slowly leading to a lower increase in blood sugar

WHOLE WHEAT

WHERE POSSIBLE, TRY TO EAT WHOLE WHEAT PASTA INSTEAD OF THE WHITE VARIETY TO KEEP YOUR BLOOD SUGAR BALANCED

WHOLE GRAIN

CHOOSE WHOLE GRAIN, SEEDED BREAD FOR MAXIMUM NUTRITION

Food swaps Instead of white bread, rice, and pasta, look for whole grain and brown versions.

DO I NEED TO TAKE SUPPLEMENTS?

At some point in your life, you are likely to have taken a nutrition supplement
or have been advised to take one. In such an unregulated industry, it can be
confusing to know what to take and if supplements are necessary at all.

———

Vitamins and minerals are essential nutrients that the body needs in very small amounts to work properly. Most of them cannot be manufactured by the body and need to come from the food we eat. Food should always come first as the preferred option for ensuring you are not deficient in any key nutrition, but sometimes our diets fall short and we may need some help—that is when supplements are useful.

IMPORTANT NUTRIENTS

For those eating a vegan diet, supplements are essential (see pp.38–39). Supplements may also be needed by plant-based eaters who are reducing animal consumption and also in times of illness, pregnancy, childhood, and old age. The nutrients required vary depending on the situation and should always be tailored to you as an individual, or you should take a sensible amount based on public health guidelines.

Health authorities around the world, especially in more northerly regions, recommend vitamin D for all ages, often 15mcg/600IU per day for everyone from 1 to 70 years old, at

which point it goes up to 20mcg/800IU (see pp.104–105). Other common supplements to look out for include iron (see pp.98–99), vitamin B12 (see pp.110–111), selenium (see pp.106–107), and iodine (see pp.108–109).

BE AWARE

Alongside evidence-based reasons for supplementing, there is now an overwhelming array of pills and concoctions on the market that are not necessary for our health. More alarmingly, when ordering online, consumers cannot always be sure that what they are purchasing in a pill or powder is of the promised quality or even the advertised ingredient. Quality can vary widely on the shelves, too, and deciphering what you need can be overwhelming. However, there are many reputable supplement companies who pay for third party certification, ensuring that their products are safe to consume.

LESS IS MORE

It's possible for supplements to interact in ways that affect one another, or to contain one or more of the same nutrients, potentially leading to toxic buildups. Less is more with supplements—they can interact with each other in positive and negative ways. For example, consuming vitamin C from food can aid iron absorption. However, when taking lots of supplements at the same time, or in a large multivitamin, the vitamins and minerals compete in the gut for absorption and one may be absorbed more effectively than another. In some cases, a multivitamin is the right choice, but in others it is not, for this reason. It is important to bear in mind that supplements are not a quick-fix solution and bioavailability of nutrients is always best from food; speaking to your health professional, a primary doctor, or registered dietitian is key.

Understanding the label

DV IS AN ABBREVIATION OF "DAILY VALUE."
DVs are set for vitamins and minerals for the purposes of food labeling and the US guidance levels on the daily amount of vitamin or mineral that the average healthy person needs to prevent deficiency. Food supplement labels list the ingredients included in the product and give the proportion of the DV value (%DV) that is contained within the supplement, for example, vitamin C, 80mg, 100% DV.

WATER-SOLUBLE VITAMINS

FAT-SOLUBLE VITAMINS

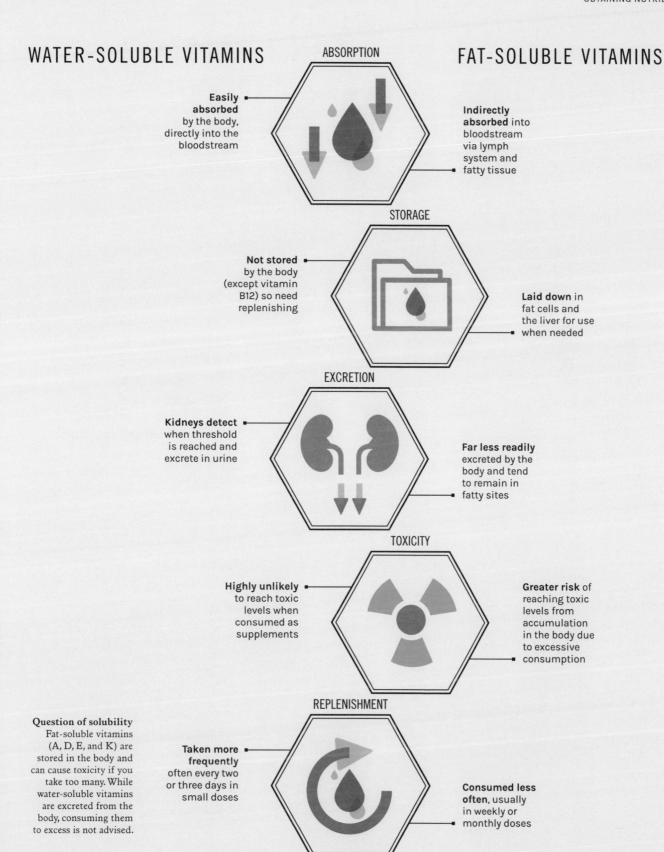

ABSORPTION

Easily absorbed by the body, directly into the bloodstream

Indirectly absorbed into bloodstream via lymph system and fatty tissue

STORAGE

Not stored by the body (except vitamin B12) so need replenishing

Laid down in fat cells and the liver for use when needed

EXCRETION

Kidneys detect when threshold is reached and excrete in urine

Far less readily excreted by the body and tend to remain in fatty sites

TOXICITY

Highly unlikely to reach toxic levels when consumed as supplements

Greater risk of reaching toxic levels from accumulation in the body due to excessive consumption

REPLENISHMENT

Question of solubility
Fat-soluble vitamins (A, D, E, and K) are stored in the body and can cause toxicity if you take too many. While water-soluble vitamins are excreted from the body, consuming them to excess is not advised.

Taken more frequently often every two or three days in small doses

Consumed less often, usually in weekly or monthly doses

WHERE CAN I FIND IRON IN A PLANT-BASED DIET?

Iron is an essential nutrient for our health and can come from many sources if you're eating a plant-based diet. Your body uses iron to make hemoglobin, a protein in red blood cells that carries oxygen from the lungs to all parts of the body, and myoglobin, a protein that provides oxygen to muscles.

IRON NEEDS

The times of your life when you need iron the most are when you are growing, during infancy, early childhood, and adolescence. Therefore, if you have a child who doesn't eat animal products, you need to be particularly aware of their iron intake. If you menstruate (have a period) or are pregnant, you may also need more iron.

PLANT-BASED IRON VS. MEAT SOURCES

Some food sources of iron are better absorbed than others. Iron from animal sources, known as heme iron, is more easily absorbed by the body than nonheme iron, which comes from plant foods. Research suggests that while vegetarians and omnivores may consume the same amounts of iron, vegetarians tend to have lower levels of iron in the blood, due to the fact that most plant sources contain oxalates and phytates, which can reduce iron absorption. Drinking tea and coffee during a meal can also have the same effect. However, there are ways to improve your iron levels while eating plant-based.

You can increase the iron absorbed from plant foods by up to four times by combining them with vitamin C. For example, you may choose a spinach salad base with berries, beans in a chili with tomatoes, or a vegetable stir-fry with peppers.

SIGNS OF DEFICIENCY

For adults and children, iron deficiency can be serious—iron deficiency results in reduced hemoglobin in red blood cells. People with mild iron deficiency may look pale, often feel tired and lacking in energy, and be more susceptible to infection. Iron supports our immune system, and a critical deficiency can produce symptoms such as heart palpitations, brittle nails, thinning hair, itchy skin (pruritus), and mouth sores or ulcers. If you experience any of these or suspect you are deficient, your doctor can test you and recommend additional supplementation.

FORTIFIED FOODS

Opting for fortified foods is another way to boost iron levels. Many foods such as baby formula and

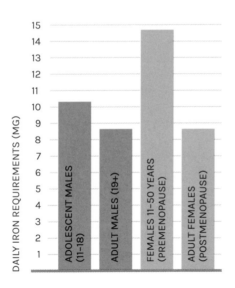

IRON NEEDS

The amount of iron needed in our daily diet varies for different groups in the population.

Iron in the body

Iron is used in the body to make hemoglobin, a protein found in red blood cells that carries oxygen from your lungs around the body.

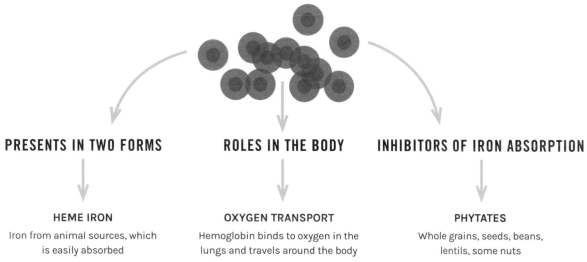

PRESENTS IN TWO FORMS

HEME IRON

Iron from animal sources, which is easily absorbed

NONHEME IRON

Iron from plant foods, which is not well absorbed but can be improved by eating with source of vitamin C

ROLES IN THE BODY

OXYGEN TRANSPORT

Hemoglobin binds to oxygen in the lungs and travels around the body

ENZYME PRODUCTION

Iron helps produce enzymes involved in many cellular processes

PROTEIN SYNTHESIS

Iron is involved in the processes that make proteins in the body

INHIBITORS OF IRON ABSORPTION

PHYTATES

Whole grains, seeds, beans, lentils, some nuts

POLYPHENOLS

Coffee, cocoa, green and black tea

CALCIUM

Dairy products, tofu

OXALIC ACID

Green tea, leafy vegetables, tea, beans, nuts, beets

bread (apart from whole grain) are fortified with iron. Often breakfast cereals have added iron, which is useful for children on plant-based diets who may not be getting their iron requirements. On Nutrition Facts labels, the amount of iron is listed as a percent (%) of the daily value. The daily value for iron is 18 mg per day. If the food has 10 to 19 percent of the daily value, it is a good source of iron.

IRON SUPPLEMENTS

If you eat a balanced and varied plant-based diet, with foods such as chickpeas, lentils, or iron-fortified breakfast cereal,s then it is likely that you are reaching your daily requirements for iron. However, in some cases, taking an iron supplement may be beneficial. This is particularly the case if you have iron deficiency anemia (IDA), a condition that affects around 30 percent of the global population. IDA can occur during pregnancy or if someone has suffered blood loss. Health guidelines suggest that those with IDA should take a form of iron supplement that contains ferrous sulfate, ferrous fumarate, or ferrous gluconate to help replenish lost stores.

CAN I GET ENOUGH CALCIUM?

Calcium isn't just needed for our bones and teeth; it is also important for our nervous system and muscular control. Dairy foods such as milk and cheese are good sources, but there are many other options if you're on a plant-based diet.

HOW MUCH CALCIUM DO I NEED?

The amount of calcium you need to take varies throughout life, and advice varies in different countries. The recommended daily amounts in the US are as follows:

- Adults 19–50 years: 1,000mg.
- Adult men 51–70 years: 1,000mg.
- Adult women 51–70 years: 1,200mg.
- Adults 71 years and older: 1,200mg.
- Pregnant/breastfeeding, 14–18 years: 1,300mg.
- Pregnant/breastfeeding, 19–50 years: 1,000mg.

SOURCES OF CALCIUM

Dark green, leafy vegetables contain high amounts of calcium. Broccoli, kale, and cabbage are all good sources of calcium, especially when eaten raw or lightly steamed (boiling vegetables can take out much of their mineral content). Calcium is sometimes added to fruit juices, soy and rice beverages, and tofu. Read product labels to find out whether a food item has added calcium. Fortified foods, including cereal, pasta, breads, and other food made with grains, may also be eaten to add calcium to your diet.

CALCIUM SUPPLEMENTS

Food first is often the best approach for nutrient absorption, but in some cases, supplementation is recommended (see pp.96–97). Some groups, such as pregnant or postmenopausal women, need more calcium. However, the amount of calcium the body absorbs from supplements differs depending on the type of

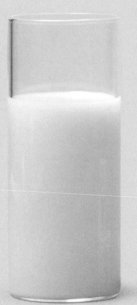

PLANT MILK

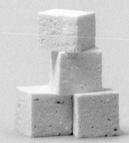

TOFU

Plant foods that contain calcium

Calcium bioavailability can be influenced by various physiological factors, such as vitamin D status, age, pregnancy, and disease, but also by the food's composition of the nutrient.

8oz CONTAINS 299mg
(23%DV) OF CALCIUM

An 8oz serving of plant-based milk will provide around 23 percent of your daily requirement.

½ CUP CONTAINS 253mg
(19%DV) OF CALCIUM

This will provide around 19 percent of the daily amount. These figures apply if the tofu is set with calcium chloride or calcium sulfate.

calcium in the supplement, how well the calcium dissolves in the intestines, and the amount of calcium in the body. The two most commonly used calcium supplement products are calcium carbonate and calcium citrate. Calcium supplements in the form of gluconate, lactate, or phosphate are also available, but they generally contain less absorbable calcium. Calcium is a nutrient where less is more, as the more you take, the less is absorbed. No more than 500mg of calcium should be taken in a single dose. If you need more than 500mg as a supplement, take the doses at least four hours apart.

BIOAVAILABILITY OF CALCIUM

Calcium can help our body function efficiently only if it is absorbed in the digestive system. Some foods help our bodies absorb calcium more efficiently. For example, vitamin D helps the absorption of calcium. Calcium sourced from plant-derived foods may be less readily absorbed because of the antinutrients known as phytates and oxalic acid that inhibit the absorption of calcium. For example, 30 percent of the calcium available from milk is absorbed by the body while only 5 percent of calcium from spinach is absorbed.

Osteoporosis

WORLDWIDE OVER 200 MILLION PEOPLE ARE LIVING WITH OSTEOPOROSIS.
This is a health condition that weakens bones, making them fragile and more likely to break. Women experiencing menopause are more vulnerable due to a reduction in estrogen, which protects bone density. Osteoporosis develops slowly over several years and is often diagnosed only when a fall or sudden impact causes a bone to break. Calcium, exercise, and vitamin D in the diet help prevent this decline in bone strength.

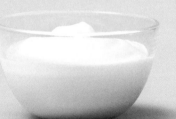

SOY YOGURT	KALE	CANNELLINI BEANS	BROCCOLI
8oz CONTAINS 344mg (27%DV) OF CALCIUM	1 CUP (RAW) CONTAINS 21mg (2%DV) OF CALCIUM	½ CUP (RAW) CONTAINS 150mg (12%DV) OF CALCIUM	½ CUP (RAW) CONTAINS 21mg (2%DV) OF CALCIUM
Soybeans are a good source of calcium because 30–40 percent of the calcium they contain is bioavailable.	Kale is a good source of plant-based calcium as it has an absorption rate of 40 percent.	The amount of calcium in cannellini beans varies slightly depending on how they are prepared.	Broccoli is a useful source of calcium and it contains vitamin C, which can also help with iron absorption.

WHY ARE OMEGA-3 FATTY ACIDS IMPORTANT?

Omega-3 is critical for the structure of our cell membranes and our brains. It makes up 40 percent of our gray matter, sperm, and cardiovascular, pulmonary, immune, and endocrine systems. Our body cannot make this essential fatty acid on its own and so we must get omega-3 from our food.

WHY IS IT IMPORTANT?

The brain is the most fat-dense organ in the body and relies heavily on omega-3 in order to carry out its everyday tasks. Research now suggests omega-3 is important as a nutrient in the diet before we are even born. Studies show those infants and children whose mothers consumed omega-3 supplements were more likely to have a higher intelligence and perform better at problem-solving tasks. There is also ongoing research looking into the reduced risk of neurodegenerative diseases and the consumption of omega-3.

TYPES OF OMEGA-3 FATTY ACIDS

The three types of omega-3 that you should be aware of are EPA (eicosapentaenoic acid), DHA (docosahexaenoic acid), and ALA (alpha-linolenic acid). EPA and DHA are mainly found in fish oils and have many health benefits, including contributing to the normal functioning of the heart, brain, and eyes. ALA (alpha-linolenic acid) is a form of omega-3 found in plant foods that the body needs to convert it to DHA and EPA before it can be used. It can, therefore, be difficult to get enough omega-3 without eating fish. The American Heart Assoiciation recommends consuming two servings of fish a week. This is believed to help prevent cardiovascular and inflammatory diseases.

SUPPLEMENTS

If you're eating a plant-based diet that doesn't contain fish, you will probably need to take an omega-3 supplement. Algae oil is a vegan option made from the algae that is the original source of DHAs and EPAs. Marine algae is very rich in omega-3 fatty acids, and fish are high in EPAs and DHAs because they eat a lot of algae. Fish oil is no longer considered the best supplement of choice as the quality of our oceans has severely declined due to sea pollution (see pp.52–53).

HOW MUCH DO WE NEED?

The daily recommendation is not to exceed 3g/day of EPA and DHA combined. In Australia, a daily intake of 160mg of EPA and DHA and 1.3g of ALA is recommended for men and 90mg of EPA and DHA and 0.8mg of ALA for women, although needs vary at different stages of life. For example, during pregnancy, childhood, and older age, omega-3 is important for brain development, growth, and health.

Omega-6

OMEGA-6 FATTY ACIDS ARE FOUND IN ALL PARTS OF THE BODY AND HELP WITH THE FUNCTION OF OUR BODY'S CELLS.

We get omega-6 from some nuts, seeds, and vegetable oils such as walnuts, hemp and sunflower seeds, and canola oil. They are good to eat in small amounts. However, we need less omega-6 than omega-3. As more of us are eating ultra-processed foods, our consumption of omega-6 fats has increased by up to 300 percent.

Types of omega-3 fatty acids

DHA and EPA are types of omega-3 fatty acids found in fish oils and algae. ALA is a type of omega-3 found in plant foods.

DHA
LONG-CHAIN POLYUNSATURATED FATTY ACIDS IN ALGAE, FISH, AND SOME NUTS AND SEEDS. IT IS IMPORTANT FOR CELLS IN THE EYES AND BRAIN

EPA
LONG-CHAIN POLYUNSATURATED FATTY ACIDS FOUND IN FISH AND ALGAE OIL. EPA IS RECOGNIZED FOR ITS ROLE IN SUPPORTING HEART HEALTH

ALA
SHORT-CHAIN POLYUNSATURATED FATTY ACIDS FOUND IN NUTS SEEDS, AND VEGETABLE OILS

Brain health
DHA is a major structural component of the brain, especially during foetal development and early infancy. It plays a crucial role in the growth and development of the nervous system. Adequate levels of DHA are important for cognitive function, memory, and overall brain health throughout life.

Eye health
DHA is a key component of the retina in the eyes. It contributes to the structure and function of the retina and is essential for maintaining healthy vision. Adequate DHA levels are particularly important during prenatal and early postnatal stages for healthy eye development in infants.

Nervous system
DHA is important for the maintenance and function of nerve cells and helps transmission of signals between nerve cells.

Mental health
EPA may have a positive effect on mental health, including conditions such as depression and anxiety.
ALA as a supplement may be effective in the prevention of Alzheimer disease progression.

Cardiovascular health
DHA, EPA, and ALA are all associated with a lower risk of heart disease.

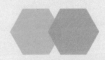

Immune system
EPA, DHA, and ALA are all believed to benefit the immune system.

Cell membrane
Both DHA and EPA are important components of cell membranes, contributing to their fluidity and stability.

Anti-inflammatory properties
DHA, EPA, and ALA have anti-inflammatory properties that contribute to overall health.

DO I NEED A VITAMIN D SUPPLEMENT?

Vitamin D plays a crucial role with our bone health, muscles, and our immune system. Most people living in the northern hemisphere are now advised to take a vitamin D supplement because of the lack of sunlight across the year.

THE SUNSHINE VITAMIN

Vitamin D is known as the sunshine vitamin because the body manufactures it by the action of sunlight on skin. It can be stored in the body and plays an important role in the absorption of the mineral calcium to build strong teeth and bones. Vitamin D is found in animal products such as fatty fish (salmon, sardines, herring, and mackerel), red meat, liver, and egg yolks. Apart from supplements, fortified foods are the biggest dietary source of vitamin D for vegans. These include orange juice, cereals, plant milks, porridge, tofu, yogurt, drinks, and some spreads. Also, some mushrooms are enriched with sunlight to store vitamin D. However, be mindful that not all mushrooms are exposed to sunlight and grown in this way, and you should read

Wild mushrooms are naturally exposed to UV light, therefore a good source of vitamin D; boost the content in supermarket mushrooms by leaving them in sunlight.

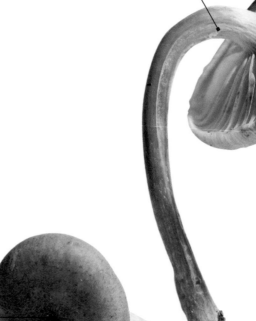

WILD MUSHROOMS MAY CONTAIN UP TO 30mcg OF VITAMIN D PER 100g, FAR MORE THAN THOSE GROWN IN THE DARK

PLANT EATERS

SOME CULTIVATED MUSHROOMS HAVE BEEN ENHANCED WITH BIOAVAILABLE VITAMIN D

Vitamin D3

Vitamin D from sunshine is inert and the body converts it into a biologically active form.

UVB DAYLIGHT

Sun exposure
UVB rays from exposure to sunlight penetrate the skin.

SKIN

Enzymes in the skin
UV light reacts with 7-dehydrocholesterol enzyme in skin cells.

PRE-VITAMIN D

Forming D3
Enzymes convert into pre-vitamin D, which restructures into D3.

VITAMIN D

Activating
Another enzyme turns D3 into calcitriol, its active form.

the packaging to check for this. You can also grow your own mushrooms and leave them on a sunny sill to absorb sunlight and store vitamin D. Some mushrooms grown in this way can store vitamin D for up to a week in the fridge.

It is unwise to try to meet your requirements from food alone because fortified foods contain vitamin D2 rather than D3. Both forms can be absorbed into the bloodstream but they are metabolized by the liver differently. The liver converts both D2 and D3 into calcifediol (also known as calcidiol), which is the main form of circulating vitamin D found in the blood, but most research suggests vitamin D3 is more effective at raising circulating vitamin D levels within the blood compared to vitamin D2.

VITAMIN D SUPPLEMENTS

The recommended daily amount of vitamin D is 400 international units (IU) for infants up to 12 months old; 600 IU for ages 1 to 70 years old; and 800 IU for those over age 70. In 2016, in the UK, it became a recommendation to introduce vitamin D supplementation to adults. Many other northern European countries, including Germany and Norway, make similar recommendations. This may be even more pertinent for those following a plant-based diet, as population studies indicate vegetarians and vegans have lower intakes of vitamin D

compared to those who consume animals and plants (omnivores). If you think you may be deficient, a blood test at your doctor's is advised, and higher doses of vitamin D may be recommended.

Those who are at risk of a deficiency tend to be older adults because as you age, your skin's ability to make vitamin D when exposed to sunlight declines. People who seldom expose their skin to sunshine may also be at risk of a deficiency.

Food sources of vitamin D

THE BEST SOURCES OF VITAMIN D ARE MEAT AND FISH-BASED. IF YOU ARE VEGAN, YOU WILL NEED TO TAKE A SUPPLEMENT.

- Mushrooms such as shiitake and maitake can contain vitamin D2 when exposed to UV light. However, the amount can vary, so it's not a reliable source.

- Fortified foods such as soy milk, cereals, and orange juice. Check the labels for more information.

- When choosing a supplement, be aware that some types of vitamin D are not vegan-friendly. Vitamin D2 is always suitable for vegans, but vitamin D3 can be derived from an animal source (such as sheep's wool) or lichen (a vegan-friendly source).

WHY IS SELENIUM IMPORTANT?

Selenium is a trace mineral that is often forgotten about but plays a key role in making our DNA and supporting our immune system. Up to one billion people around the world are said to be deficient in this mineral.

Meats, eggs, and seafood contain high amounts of selenium, while Brazil nuts, whole wheat bread, whole grains such as brown rice, legumes including lentils, spinach, broccoli, mushrooms, and garlic are plant sources. The micronutrient selenium is essential for processes involving the thyroid gland (see pp.108–109) and the reproductive system. It is also used in DNA synthesis and protects from oxidative damage and infection. Once consumed, selenium is incorporated into proteins that primarily function as antioxidants, keeping cells in the body healthy and free from damage. Research suggests that selenium may also be associated with cognitive functioning, and it is thought to have anti-inflammatory effects and support immune function, including antiviral protection. One of selenium's critical roles in human health is its incorporation into selenoproteins, a type of protein synthesized within the body. These proteins integrate ingested selenium into their basic structure, therefore giving rise to their name. Selenoproteins are involved in a

magnitude of vital biological functions within the body such as antioxidant defense, skeletal muscle regeneration, cell maintenance, thyroid hormone metabolism, immune responses, and reproduction. These functions are critical for your overall health, and without adequate selenium intake, your body is at risk of becoming incapable of maintaining them. This places you at an increased risk of a number of chronic diseases, such as cancer, inflammatory disorders, cardiovascular disease, and impairment of bone mineralization, reduced fertility, and impaired thyroid function.

SELENIUM DEFICIENCY

If you are deficient in selenium, you may experience infertility, muscle weakness, fatigue, mental fog, hair loss, and a weakened immune system. When following a vegan or plant-based diet, it is important to ensure that you are consuming dietary forms of selenium and to be aware that a supplement may be required. Absorption of this mineral can be affected

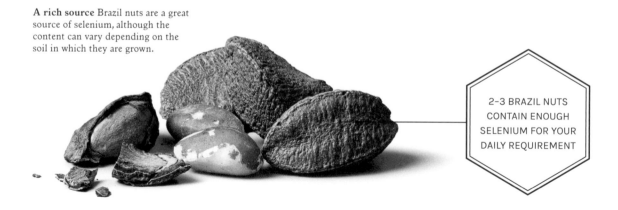

A rich source Brazil nuts are a great source of selenium, although the content can vary depending on the soil in which they are grown.

2-3 BRAZIL NUTS CONTAIN ENOUGH SELENIUM FOR YOUR DAILY REQUIREMENT

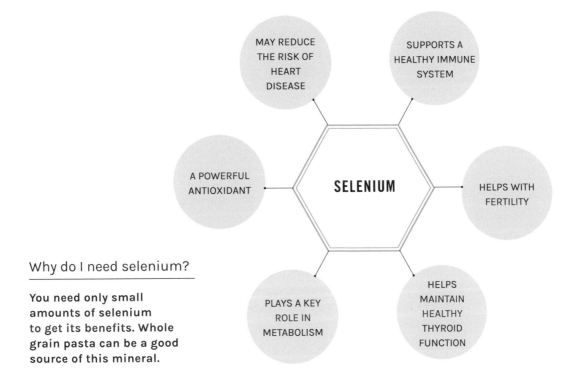

Why do I need selenium?

You need only small amounts of selenium to get its benefits. Whole grain pasta can be a good source of this mineral.

by digestive disorders such as Crohn's disease or if you have HIV or are undergoing dialysis. Others who need to be particularly careful about whether they are getting enough selenium are those who are pregnant, have thyroid disease, cancer, and weakened immune functioning.

SOIL AND SELENIUM

The amount of selenium found in plant foods varies depending upon the soil where it is grown. As this is not something you can determine when buying food, it is best to eat a wide variety of plant foods to ensure you're getting enough of this mineral. This amount is influenced by the geographical location and the geological properties (such as the bedrock upon which the soil is situated) of the area in which the crops are grown. The overall selenium concentration of a crop is determined by the complex interaction of a number of factors and is not just simply determined by the quantity found within the soil.

Soil pH levels affect the form of selenium available to plants. The most soluble and bioavailable form of selenium to plants is selenate. Alkaline soil more readily oxidizes selenium into this favored form for absorption than acidic soil, and it is then taken up through the roots of the plant. The form of selenium in the soil is determined by the presence of organic matter, which determines the microbial activity of the soil. Microorganisms play a vital role in transforming inorganic forms of selenium into the organic, plant-absorbable forms. This conversion enhances the availability of selenium for plant uptake and therefore selenium accumulates in the crop.

As selenate is the more absorbable form of selenium, it is favored by plants for its uptake. Selenite is an inorganic form of selenium and is also present in soil but must undergo a chemical conversion before it can be taken up by the roots of the plant. This conversion is determined by the microbial activity of the soil, which is first influenced by the soils' organic matter content.

SHOULD I BE CONSCIOUS OF IODINE INTAKE?

Iodine deficiency impacts 2 billion people around the world with rates rising in the West, especially in adolescent women and pregnant women. We need this trace mineral for growth and development as it plays a key role in our cognition.

SOURCES OF IODINE

Iodine comes from the soil and the ocean, and levels in our food varies due to the farming practices in use and the season. It is especially important if you are eating a plant-based or vegan diet to be aware of this nutrient as the most common source tends to be dairy foods, fish, meat, eggs, and shellfish. Vegetables may have a small trace of iodine but are generally regarded as a poor source of the nutrient. Seaweed is understood to be one of the most potent sources of iodine, such that one sheet of nori seaweed (used to make sushi) can contain up to ⅓ of your recommended daily intake. With this in mind, you should be aware of your iodine intake as it can be easy to consume far more than the recommended amount, which can have negative effects on your thyroid gland. Iodine may be added to plant-based milk alternatives and other food items—check the label. In some countries, including the US, a variety of foods are fortified with salt containing iodine, although adding too much salt to our diet is not recommended. Some research explored adding iodine to fruits and vegetables for a more healthy alternative, but this is not common practice.

WHY DO WE NEED IODINE?

Iodine regulates metabolism, and a deficiency can cause lack of growth and development. It is particularly important for women planning a pregnancy, those who are pregnant, and infants to ensure healthy brain development and cognitive

Signs of hypothyroidism

If you have an iodine deficiency, it may cause hypothyroidism—when the thyroid gland doesn't produce enough hormones to meet the body's needs.

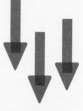

FATIGUE AND LETHARGY

Persistent tiredness and fatigue caused by a lower metabolic rate can be a sign of hypothyroidism.

skills. Iodine is also needed for thyroid hormones—they cannot work well without enough of this nutrient, and a deficiency leads to an underactive or overactive thyroid gland.

Others who may be at risk of deficiency are those who, in addition to not consuming enough iodine, consume foods containing goitrogens. These are substances that can inhibit the way the body uses iodine and are found in some foods such as broccoli, Brussels sprouts, and soy.

HOW MUCH?

As a general rule, the daily recommendation is 150mcg of iodine per day, but this varies at different times of life. For example, when pregnant and breastfeeding, there is an increased requirement of 220mcg to 290mcg to ensure the thyroid hormone production in the fetus or baby is working, to balance any potential losses from the mother, and to supply the fetus with iodine so it can produce its own thyroid hormones after thyroid onset midgestation. If a pregnant woman does not get enough iodine in pregnancy, this may impact the development of the baby's brain and impact the child's IQ later in life, so it is crucial to ensure you meet your daily intake if planning a pregnancy.

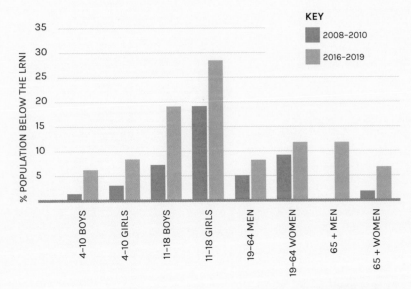

KEY
- 2008–2010
- 2016–2019

% POPULATION BELOW THE LRNI

4-10 BOYS / 4-10 GIRLS / 11-18 BOYS / 11-18 GIRLS / 19-64 MEN / 19-64 WOMEN / 65 + MEN / 65 + WOMEN

IODINE SUPPLEMENTS

Vegans and vegetarians are likely to need additional support from a supplement. During pregnancy, check the supplement does not exceed 150mcg as the rest of the requirement will probably come from your diet. Seaweed or kelp supplements may provide a dangerous amount of iodine, so check with a healthcare professional before taking them.

IODINE INTAKES

The number of people below the LRNI (lower reference nutrient intake), meaning they are not absorbing enough iodine has grown between 2008–2019.

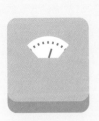

GAIN IN WEIGHT

Hypothyroidism can slow down your metabolism, leading to weight gain. Thyroid hormones are key to metabolic rate.

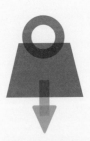

WEAKNESS

Thyroid hormones are required to regulate muscle function and energy metabolism. Insufficient levels could result in weakness.

SENSITIVITY TO COLD

Reduced thyroid hormone levels can impact thermoregulatory processes, reducing heat generation and retention.

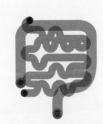

CONSTIPATION

Hypothyroidism can slow the digestive processes in the gastrointestinal tract, leading to constipation.

WHY DO WE NEED VITAMIN B12?

Vitamin B12 is found naturally only in animal products. If you are eating some meat and dairy, you are probably getting enough B12, but if you are vegan, you will need to supplement. It is estimated that up to 15 percent of the general population has a vitamin B12 deficiency

---

WHAT IS B12?

Vitamin B12, otherwise known as cobalamin, plays an important role in our red blood cells, DNA, nervous system, and brain development. In order to be absorbed, this vitamin binds itself to the proteins we eat, separates in the stomach with our stomach acid, and then goes on to bind again with another protein to help with absorption in the intestines.

Without enough B12, you are at risk of impacting many areas of your health, especially your heart and brain health. This is owed to the role B12 plays in breaking down homocysteine, a protein in our bodies that is linked to an increased risk of heart

disease and stroke. This does not mean supplements of B vitamins reduce risk of heart disease, though (see pp.190–191), as heart disease can be caused by many different factors.

DO'S AND DON'TS

There are quite a few myths circulating around plant-based sources of B12—they don't exist! Spirulina is not a source of vitamin B12, nori (the seaweed) may have traces but not enough to be considered a source, and those who eat a vegan diet will not get enough from consuming nutritional yeast alone. Nutritional yeast doesn't contain B12

Breaking down homocysteine

B12 plays a key role in converting homocysteine back into methionine, and deficiencies in B12 can lead to elevated homocysteine levels. Homocysteine is an amino acid produced by the breakdown of methionine, a building block for proteins in the body.

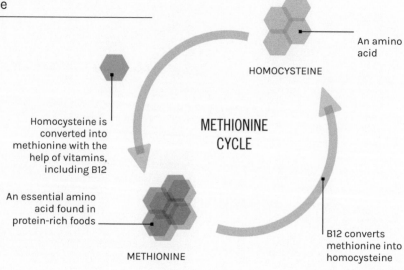

An amino acid

HOMOCYSTEINE

Homocysteine is converted into methionine with the help of vitamins, including B12

METHIONINE CYCLE

An essential amino acid found in protein-rich foods

B12 converts methionine into homocysteine

METHIONINE

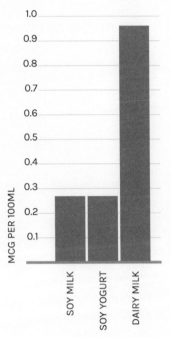

B12 LEVELS

Cow's milk contains much higher levels of vitamin B12 than unfortified plant alternatives.

unless it is fortified with the vitamin, so always check the label. The best option for plant-eaters who do not consume any or enough animal produce is to add fortified foods into the diet and to take a nutritional supplement containing B12. This is particularly important for anyone who is pregnant and eating a plant-based diet because the fetus needs vitamin B12 for neurologic development, and a deficiency can lead to permanent neurological damage (see pp.160–161).

A type of anemia called pernicious anemia can be caused by a B12 deficiency, although this is not due to dietary intake. It can occur when an autoimmune disease attacks and harms gut cells, resulting in the destructions of cells that produce intrinsic factor, a protein needed so that the body can absorb vitamin B12. Even a supplement of a very high dose cannot solve the problem. Injections of B12 may be required and the condition must be monitored by a health professional.

B12 DEFICIENCIES

When checking levels of B12, blood tests are not always an accurate measure. It is important to see a qualified health professional who can assess other markers in a blood test to check for a vitamin B12 deficiency. Signs of deficiency may include:

● Megaloblastic anemia—a condition of larger than normal sized red blood cells and a smaller than normal amount; this occurs because there is not enough vitamin B12 in the diet or poor absorption

● Pernicious anemia—a type of megaloblastic anemia caused by a lack of intrinsic factor so that vitamin B12 is not absorbed

● Fatigue, weakness

● Nerve damage with numbness, tingling in the hands and legs

● Memory loss, confusion

● Depression

● Seizures

GETTING THE RIGHT B12 SUPPLEMENT

Choosing a B12 supplement that works for you is important. Some come in very high doses, which is unnecessary and doesn't guarantee you will absorb the B12 you need. Absorption is dependent on your unique makeup and how much intrinsic factor you have. If you have a severe deficiency, such as pernicious anemia, your doctor will often prescribe injections into the muscle. Please speak to a health professional before taking a supplement.

WILL I GET ENOUGH ZINC?

You need only small amounts of this trace mineral, but what we do require is crucial for our chemical reactions inside our bodies, from the formation of our DNA to healing damaged tissue; building protein, reproductive systems, and fertility; and supporting our immune systems.

WHY DO WE NEED ZINC?

More than 300 different enzymes use zinc to carry out essential chemical processes in the body, including immune cell development and function, the creation of DNA, the replication, damage repair of cells, and protein synthesis, specifically collagen. Zinc also impacts our skin health and our ability to heal wounds.

If you are eating a plant-based diet, it is important to be aware of your zinc intake as foods like whole grains have lower bioavailability of the mineral than animal foods. The World Health Organization (WHO) recommends that plant-based eaters should aim for more than three times the zinc intake of those eating a diet containing meat and dairy. So women should aim for 8mg (12–13mg if pregnant or breastfeeding), and men should aim for 11mg for optimal health. Those who are vegan are most likely to be deficient in zinc—in one study, 76 percent of vegan subjects had intakes below recommended amounts. Some meat substitutes, such as mycoprotein (Quorn), have been shown to

The power of phytates

Phytates are compounds that are naturally present in plants. Some foods that contain more phytates can reduce the amount of minerals you may absorb. If you eat a range of plant foods every week, you should absorb enough essential minerals for good health.

FOOD LOW IN PHYTATES

Beneficial role
Foods lower in phytates and their phytate content:

MILLET
(0.18%-1.67%)

CHICKPEAS
(0.28%-1.6%)

LENTILS
(0.27%-1.51%)

OATS
(0.42%-1.16%)

FOODS RICH IN PHYTATES

Lower mineral absorption
Foods that may hinder the absorption of minerals and their phytate content:

ALMONDS
(0.35%-9.42%)

WALNUTS
(0.2%-6.69%)

KIDNEY BEANS
(0.61%-2.38%)

CORN
(6.39%)

be a valuable source of zinc for plant-based eaters in several studies and worth including in plant-based diets (see pp.122–123). While zinc deficiency is rare, our requirements do increase during pregnancy and breastfeeding and can be trickier to obtain as we age. Men need to be aware of getting enough zinc because it supports healthy sperm (see pp.180–181).

If following a sustainable diet that incorporates small amounts of meat and a wealth of zinc-containing plant-foods, then you should be getting an adequate amount of this mineral.

ZINC ABSORPTION

It is important to note the absorption of zinc from some plant foods such as legumes and whole grains can be impaired by the phytates they contain, but if you consume a large amount and a variety of these foods, this shouldn't impact your overall intake. Some research points toward eating fermented plant foods for zinc as the fermentation process can help remove the phytates and enable more zinc to be available to your body (see pp.78–79). Other methods such as canning, soaking, and sprouting may also be helpful in aiding zinc absorption.

Zinc as a skin treatment

ZINC OXIDE WAS USED IN OINTMENTS TO TREAT WOUNDS, AS NOTED IN ANCIENT GREEK MEDICAL TEXTS.

Today, zinc oxide is still a popular over-the-counter skin treatment. It may defend against sunburn by reflecting and scattering ultraviolet rays so they do not penetrate the skin. It is also used to treat inflamed skin conditions like burns, eczema, bedsores, and diaper rash. The compound forms a protective barrier on the skin's surface, repelling away moisture and allowing the skin to heal. It may also aid enzymes to break down damaged collagen tissue so that new tissue can be formed. No negative side effects have been reported, although you should check with a doctor before using zinc in this way.

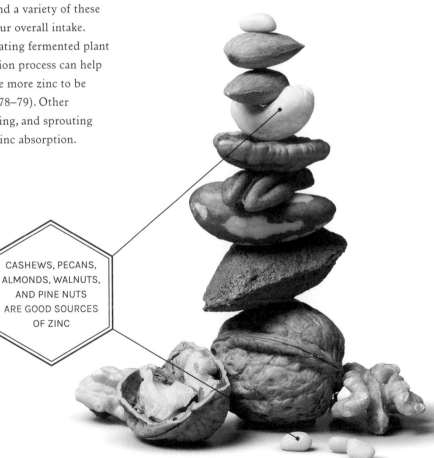

CASHEWS, PECANS, ALMONDS, WALNUTS, AND PINE NUTS ARE GOOD SOURCES OF ZINC

Nuts are a useful addition to a plant-based diet to make sure you're getting enough zinc on a weekly basis.

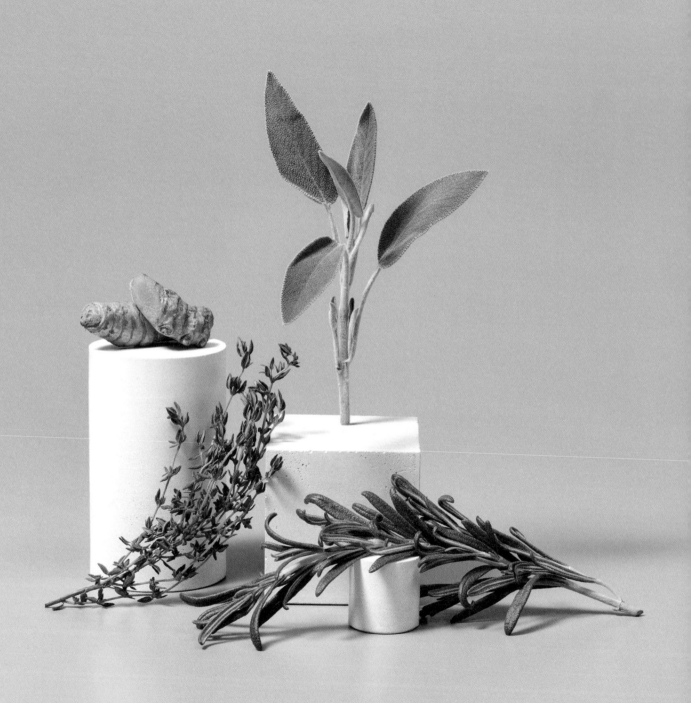

PLANT-BASED COOKING AND SHOPPING

WHAT ASPECTS OF FLAVOR AND TEXTURE MIGHT I MISS IF I GO PLANT-BASED?

If you are thinking about changing your diet from one containing meat to a plant-based one, you may be wondering how to recreate the taste and flavor of your favorite animal products. There are many ways that you can still enjoy flavorful, pleasingly textured food without eating meat.

———————

Change isn't easy for human beings. In fact, part of the brain, the amygdala, interprets change as a threat and releases the hormones for fear, fight, or flight. However, change can also be beneficial, helping you grow and explore new things. Changing something as fundamental as your diet in a major way is a big shift, and so it is understandable that you may be worried about whether you'll still enjoy eating in the same way as before. Many people are perhaps put off by the concept of plant-based eating based on their enjoyment of the appearance, flavor, texture, and mouthfeel of animal-based products. When we

eat meat and dairy foods, they give us a sense of fullness, possibly due to their fat content and rich umami flavor. However, there are now plant-based alternatives to match these qualities.

TASTE

Research shows that taste plays the most important role in whether people like meat substitutes. Some consumers refuse to purchase protein alternatives because they "won't like the taste." Taste is a major driver in favor of meat, and it is a challenge for the food industry to match the flavor of meat alternatives with regular meat. Interestingly, consumers find plant-based alternatives more convincing when they imitate processed meat products (hamburgers, sausages, and nuggets) than when they imitate unprocessed meats (for example, steak). This may be because the texture of processed meats is easier to replicate than unprocessed meat.

TEXTURE

To mimic the sensory properties of meat, plant proteins require a high degree of processing and manipulation, which modifies the product to such a

Chart

| | 40 | 30 | 20 | 10 | 0 |

Categories (x-axis):
- Trying to lose weight
- Watching my cholesterol
- Concerns about animal welfare
- Worried about eating too much saturated fat
- Someone in my household is vegetarian or vegan

MOVING AWAY FROM MEAT

A survey showed that more Millenials than other age groups are eating meat alternatives for health and animal welfare reasons.

KEY

▮ Millenials

▮ Non-Millenials

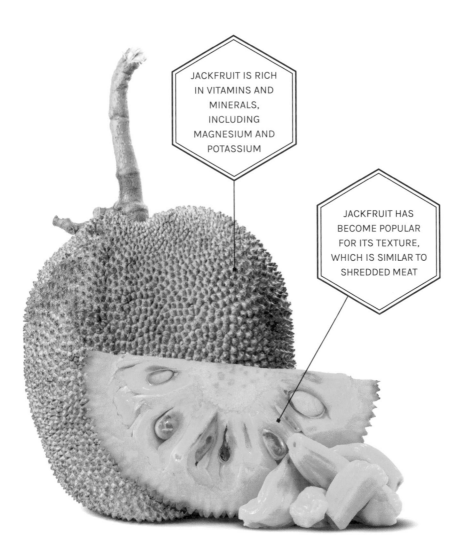

JACKFRUIT IS RICH IN VITAMINS AND MINERALS, INCLUDING MAGNESIUM AND POTASSIUM

JACKFRUIT HAS BECOME POPULAR FOR ITS TEXTURE, WHICH IS SIMILAR TO SHREDDED MEAT

THE PLANT-BASED MEAT ALTERNATIVES GLOBAL MARKET IS PROJECTED TO REACH $3.5 BILLION BY 2026

IN A US SURVEY, TWO-THIRDS OF PARTICIPANTS SAID THEY HAD REDUCED THEIR MEAT CONSUMPTION IN THE LAST THREE YEARS

40%
OF CONSUMERS WORLDWIDE ARE TRYING TO REDUCE THEIR CONSUMPTION OF ANIMAL PROTEINS

degree from the original ingredients that it can trigger food neophobia (a reluctance to try new foods). Ultra-processed food eaten regularly is bad for our health, and vegan foods are no exception (see pp.60–61). Data collected from a survey in the US found the main reasons for not increasing the consumption of protein alternatives were that they were "too processed" (45 percent of consumers) and "high in sodium" (42 percent of consumers) among the group unlikely to purchase them.

MEAT SUBSTITUTES

If you are missing the flavor and texture of cheese, meat, and other dairy products, there are many ways that you can add them to your meals without using animal products. For example, if you miss cheese, you can use fortified plant-based cheese alternatives or nutritional yeast (see pp.124–125). For a meaty texture, you might try jackfruit, a tropical tree fruit used to recreate pulled-pork dishes. There are a number of ways of adding creaminess to your cooking without milk or cream (see pp.146–147).

There are many meat substitute products now available. Research shows that those who consume a vegetarian and vegan diet are more likely to accept plant-based alternatives that lack the smell and texture of meat than omnivores and flexitarians, who prefer alternatives that resemble meat.

WHAT ARE TOFU AND TEMPEH?

Tofu and tempeh are incredibly nutrient-rich sources of protein to include in your diet and can be useful if you're eating plant-based. They are both made with soybeans but are processed in different ways.

Tofu is an ancient food made from soy milk that was first produced in China more than 2,000 years ago. It remains a staple of Chinese cooking today. Soy milk is made by soaking, blending, straining, and boiling soybeans. It is then condensed and pressed into blocks. Different kinds of tofu are distinguished by their firmness and texture, ranging from silken to firm; there are also smoked and flavored varieties.

Tempeh was developed in Indonesia around 300 years ago and is made using soybeans that are fermented, soaked, hulled, and then cooked until they form a firm block. The fermentation process adds to its texture and distinctive flavor. Although both tofu and tempeh are processed food items, they are beneficial to your health. Out of the two options, tempeh is slightly less processed than tofu, although they are both nutritionally similar. Neither have much flavor of their own, but they are good at absorbing others, have a chewy texture similar to meat, hold up to cooking at high heats, and will crisp up well. Both are a source of complete protein and may also contain other important nutrients.

For example, some tofu can be a source of calcium if it is calcium-set.

SOY AND MENOPAUSE

The research surrounding soy is largely positive, and it's believed that it is particularly beneficial for women going through menopause. Plant compounds called phytoestrogens found in soy may help ease hot flashes and night sweats. So far, research has focused on one type: isoflavones, found in soybeans and soy-based foods and drinks. Only 10–20 percent of Asian women (who have a large intake of soy) experience hot flashes compared with a majority of perimenopausal or menopausal women in the US, where soy intake is much lower.

Scientists don't yet understand the precise mechanism, but isoflavones appear to produce a weak estrogen-like effect without affecting estrogen levels. Soy isoflavones have a slightly different chemical structure to human estrogen and affect people in different ways. Some people may experience mild estrogen-like effects such as less severe hot flashes, while others feel no effects.

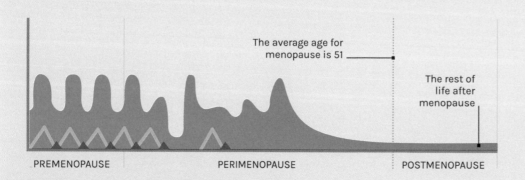

The average age for menopause is 51

The rest of life after menopause

PREMENOPAUSE   PERIMENOPAUSE   POSTMENOPAUSE

KEY

■ Estrogen levels

▲ Menstrual period

▬ Progesterone levels

MENOPAUSE TRANSITION

The symptoms of this transition can last for many years during perimenopause.

HOW MUCH SOY SHOULD I HAVE?

EATING TWO SERVINGS OR AROUND 50mg OF ISOFLAVONES (A TYPE OF PHYTOESTROGEN FOUND IN SOY) PER DAY IS ASSOCIATED WITH REDUCED FREQUENCY AND SEVERITY OF HOT FLASHES. THE FOLLOWING CONTAIN 50mg OF ISOFLAVONES:

3.5oz (100g) SOY CRUMBLES

3.5oz (100g) TEMPEH

3.5oz (100g) EDAMAME BEANS

2 x 8oz (250ml) SOY DRINKS

1 x 8oz (250ml) SOY DRINK AND

7oz (200g) PLAIN SOY YOGURT ALTERNATIVE

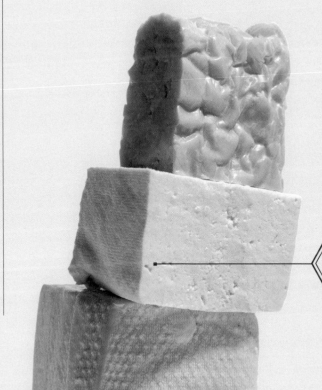

TOFU
FIRM TOFU IS USEFUL IN DISHES SUCH AS KEBABS OR IN PLACE OF MARINATED MEAT

TEMPEH
THIS IS GREAT IN STIR-FRIES AND CAN BE GRILLED OR BARBECUED OR SLICED AND EATEN IN SANDWICHES

SOY FOODS ARE RICH IN NUTRIENTS, INCLUDING B VITAMINS, FIBER, POTASSIUM, AND MAGNESIUM

SOY IS A COMPLETE PROTEIN

SOY'S ANTIOXIDANT AND ANTI-INFLAMMATORY EFFECTS MAY REDUCE THE OXIDATIVE STRESSES ASSOCIATED WITH ALZHEIMER'S DISEASE AND PARKINSON'S DISEASE

Tofu and tempeh These foods may have benefits for those going through menopause.

WHAT IS SEITAN?

Seitan is a vegan alternative to meat made using wheat so is not useful for those with gluten intolerances. A more recent innovation than tofu or tempeh, it is often used to make alternatives to bacon and deli meat, and you can make it at home.

WHAT IS GLUTEN?

Seitan is made from wheat gluten flour and water or broth and has a dense and rubbery texture. The proteins found in wheat and several other grains, including rye and barley, are gluten-forming proteins. Gluten is a composite of two proteins: gliadin and glutenin. When the grains are made into flour and water is added to create a dough, these two proteins combine to create an elastic texture, which allows bread to develop its flexible, airy structure. The word "gluten" is similar to "glue," and it quite literally holds or glues the dough together. This is why it works so well as a meat alternative in seitan—the texture is very chewy when cooked.

In addition to wheat, rye, and barley, gluten is also found in spelt, durum, emmer, semolina, farina, farro, graham, khorasan wheat, einkorn, and triticale (a blend of wheat and rye). Oats—although naturally gluten-free—often contain gluten from cross-contamination when they are grown near, or processed in, the same location as the grains listed above.

Some people react badly to gluten when their body senses it as a toxin, causing their immune cells to overreact and attack it. While some people are intolerant or sensitive to gluten, around 1 percent of the population have celiac disease, an autoimmune disorder, which is more serious (see pp.200–201).

Gluten isn't inherently bad; it is incredibly useful and is a problem only for those who cannot tolerate it. For those who are intolerant, it is also important not to rely on processed gluten-free foods that may be high in calories, sugar, saturated fat, and salt and low in nutrients. These foods may include gluten-free cookies, bars, and chips. Often they are made with processed unfortified rice, tapioca, corn, or potato flours, and do not contain the protein gluten does.

MAKING YOUR OWN SEITAN

You can buy seitan, although it could be difficult to find in some mainstream supermarkets compared to other plant-based meat alternatives. Lots of ready-made options also contain additional salt/sodium or additives to extend shelf life, so you may prefer to make your own with added herbs and spices for extra flavor.

There are two main techniques to create seitan. Using the flour washing method, you make a dough ball with flour and water. You then knead the dough ball under water to "wash" out the starches. The wheat starch in flour is water-soluble, so when the dough ball is kneaded and washed under water, the starch is released into the water. You can then flatten out the seitan and cook it in vegetable stock. Then leave it in the fridge overnight before using in

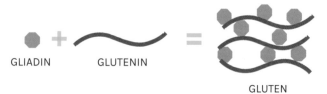

GLIADIN   GLUTENIN   GLUTEN

Gluten formation The proteins gliadin and glutenin combine with water to create a mesh structure known as gluten, which has an elastic quality that is especially useful in baking.

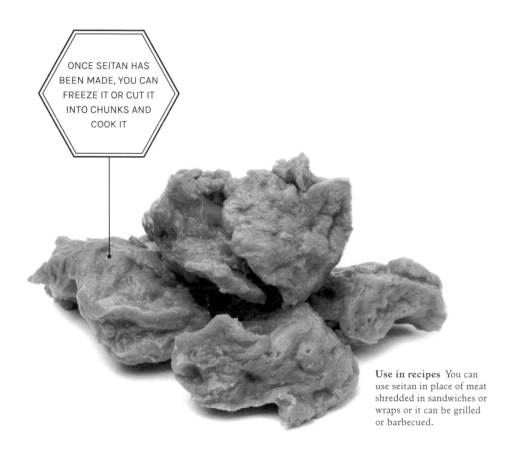

ONCE SEITAN HAS
BEEN MADE, YOU CAN
FREEZE IT OR CUT IT
INTO CHUNKS AND
COOK IT

Use in recipes You can
use seitan in place of meat
shredded in sandwiches or
wraps or it can be grilled
or barbecued.

ENVIRONMENTAL IMPACT:

A SURVEY BASED
ON UK SEITAN
PRODUCTS FOUND
THAT THERE WAS

46.6kg

OF CO_2 EMISSIONS
FOR EVERY 100kg
OF SEITAN

COMPARED TO
6,000kg

FOR EVERY 100kg
OF **BEEF**

a recipe. The other method is slightly easier as it uses vital wheat gluten—a wheat flour dough that is already washed to remove the starch. It is pure gluten and is made of about 80 percent protein.

HOW TO EAT SEITAN

Traditionally, wheat proteins like seitan are used widely in Japan, Korea, China, and Russia to replace beef or chicken. Gluten has the capacity to form a thin film when stretched, resulting in a naturally stringy structure, which helps seitan to imitate the texture and consistency of meat well. Often dubbed as "high protein," although it doesn't have a complete amino acid profile, the specific nutrition provided by seitan depends on the kind of wheat flour or vital wheat gluten that is used, how it is made, and the amount of water or broth used.

Fructans

A LOT OF PROCESSED BREADS THAT CONTAIN GLUTEN ALSO CONTAIN FRUCTANS, WHICH SOME PEOPLE HAVE PROBLEMS PROCESSING.
Some people might think they have a gluten intolerance when in fact they are sensitive to fructans. A fructan is a molecule consisting of a chain of fructose molecules joined together, and with a glucose molecule at the end. Fructans are sugars that are included in the FODMAP group of carbohydrates that can cause digestive disorders. It can be difficult to find out what triggers you have if you have a food sensitivity. This is why it is important to work alongside a FODMAP-trained health professional (see pp.82-83).

WHAT IS MYCOPROTEIN?

High in fiber and low in saturated fat, mycoprotein is a meat substitute made from a fungus. In the 1960s, the question of the future of food availability was surfacing. After testing 3,000 microorganisms taken from soil samples around the world, fungus was found to be a suitable base for a meat substitute.

———————

Mycoprotein is sold under the name "Quorn." The main ingredient of Quorn mycoprotein is *Fusarium venenatum*, an ascomycete, which is a type of fungus that naturally occurs in the soil.

HOW IS IT MADE?

To make mycoprotein, the fungus is fermented in a controlled environment to create a biomass of protein-rich cells. These are processed to remove excess water, then texture is added to create a meatlike substance. Flavors and seasoning are added, and the substance is formed into a range of products, including burger patties, crumbles, pieces, fillets, and nuggets. Some products have egg added so check the labels if you're vegan or have allergies. The process has a reduced carbon and water footprint relative to beef and chicken. In fact, Quorn mycoprotein production uses 95 percent less CO_2 than typical ground beef. The carbon footprint of Quorn mycoprotein is 40 times lower than the global average for beef and six times lower than the global average for chicken. The water footprint of Quorn mycoprotein is 30 times lower than the global average for beef and six times lower than the global average for chicken. Quorn is a sustainable source of protein that could help feed growing populations.

HEALTH BENEFITS

Mycoprotein is nutritious, but if you are using it to replace red meat such as ground beef, remember that it does not contain iron. Consuming mycoprotein instead of meat can help maintain healthy blood cholesterol levels, promote muscle synthesis, control glucose and insulin levels, and increase a feeling of fullness or satiety (due to its fiber and protein).

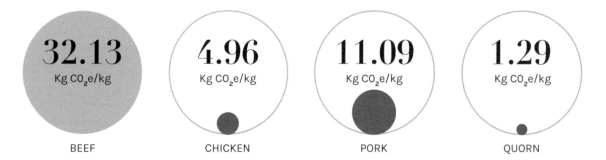

32.13 Kg CO_2e/kg — BEEF

4.96 Kg CO_2e/kg — CHICKEN

11.09 Kg CO_2e/kg — PORK

1.29 Kg CO_2e/kg — QUORN

Comparison of different proteins These figures represents the carbon footprints of different proteins and Quorn.

KEY NUTRITION (PER 100g)

THESE FIGURES COMPARE NUTRITIONAL VALUES FOR QUORN CRUMBLES AND CHICKEN BY WEIGHT.

QUORN	CHICKEN (COOKED)
ENERGY: 94.0 KCAL	ENERGY: 165 KCAL
PROTEIN: 14.5g	PROTEIN: 31g
CARBS: 4.5g	CARBS: 0g
FAT: 2.0g (OF WHICH SATURATED: 0.5g)	FAT: 3.6g (OF WHICH SATURATED: 1g)
FIBER: 5.3g	FIBER: 0g

Ways to use mycoprotein:

MYCOPROTEIN (SOLD AS QUORN) IS A USEFUL SOURCE OF PROTEIN THAT CAN BE USED TO REPLACE MEAT IN MANY CLASSIC FAMILY RECIPES

SHEPHERD'S PIE AND BOLOGNESE

USE QUORN CRUMBLES INSTEAD OF GROUND BEEF OR LAMB IN THESE DISHES AND IT WILL ABSORB THE RICH FLAVORS OF THE SAUCE

GRAIN BOWL

ADD QUORN TO QUINOA OR MIX WITH GREENS AND VEGGIES TO ADD PROTEIN TO YOUR GRAIN BOWL FOR A NUTRITIOUS LUNCH

CURRY AND PAELLA

ADD QUORN PIECES TO A FLAVORFUL CURRY SAUCE OR MIX QUORN STRIPS INTO A PAELLA BURSTING WITH INFUSED RICE AND VEGETABLES.

FILLETS

TRY GRILLING, SAUTÉING, OR BAKING QUORN FILLETS IN A RANGE OF DISHES FROM STIR-FRIES TO SALADS.

QUORN FILLETS

THESE ARE A VERSATILE FORM OF MYCOPROTEIN AND CAN BE USED TO REPLACE CHICKEN IN MANY RECIPES

QUORN CRUMBLES

EAT THIS WITH BEANS AND PULSES TO BOOST THE PROTEIN AND IRON CONTENT OF YOUR DISH

Mycoprotein is a versatile form of plant-based protein that is available in many forms and can easily be incorporated into a range of different meals.

WHAT IS NUTRITIONAL YEAST?

Also known as nooch, nutritional yeast is a deactivated yeast that can be used to add flavor and nutrients to a plant-based diet. It has a savory, nutty flavor and is a useful source of protein for plant-based eaters.

Nutritional yeast is made using yeast cells, which are grown for several days in a sugar-rich medium such as glucose, often from either sugar cane or beet molasses. When the yeast is ready, it is deactivated with heat and then harvested, washed, dried, and packaged ready to use in cooking or seasoning to give a savory or umami flavor to dishes. Umami is one of the five basic tastes. It has been described as savory and is characteristic of broths and cooked meats. People experience umami through taste receptors that respond to glutamates (amino acids) and nucleotides (molecules that store and transfer genetic information), which are found in meat broths and fermented products. You will see nutritional yeast sold as either powder, granules, or as yellow flakes, and it is often located in the same aisle of the supermarket as herbs and spices.

WHAT ARE THE BENEFITS?

Nutritional yeast can be classified into fortified yeast and nonfortified yeast. Both types provide iron, but fortified yeast provides 20 percent of your daily recommended intake, while unfortified yeast provides only 5 percent. Unfortified nutritional yeast provides 35–100 percent of vitamins B1 and B2. There is some confusion about the source of vitamin B12 in nutritional yeast, as nutritional yeast is often used by vegans who want to supplement their diet with vitamin B12. Yeast cannot produce vitamin B12. Vitamin B12 is naturally produced only by some bacteria. Some, but not all, brands of nutritional yeast are fortified with vitamin B12. When fortified, vitamin B12 (usually cyanocobalamin) is produced separately and added to the yeast.

Nutritional yeast is a great source of high-quality protein because it contains all nine essential amino acids (see pp.92–93). Many people on a vegan or plant-based diet do not consume enough vitamin B12, which is a vital nutrient for keeping blood and nerve cells healthy (see pp.110–111). Opt for fortified versions that are especially rich in B vitamins. Check the label to make sure the yeast includes thiamine (B1), riboflavin (B2), niacin (B3), B6, and B12, as well as potassium, iron, and other

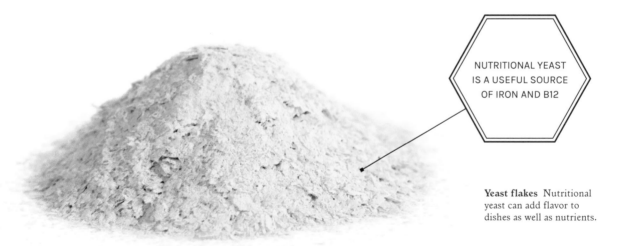

NUTRITIONAL YEAST
IS A USEFUL SOURCE
OF IRON AND B12

Yeast flakes Nutritional yeast can add flavor to dishes as well as nutrients.

trace minerals. Nutritional values vary depending on the brand you purchase and the form the nutritional yeast comes in. Nutritional yeast is also naturally low in sodium and calories, and it's fat-free, sugar-free, gluten-free, and vegan.

HOW CAN I USE NUTRITIONAL YEAST?

Nutritional yeast is a useful addition to plant-based recipes and can be sprinkled over the top of the finished dish or added as an ingredient. Some meals that you can add nutritional yeast to are vegan macaroni and cheese and lentil and veggie pasta bake; it can also be used to add flavor to salads, soups, marinades, sauces, and smoothies.

Nutritional yeast is often confused with Baker's yeast and Brewer's yeast as they are made from the same species of yeast, *Saccharomyces cerevisiae*. However, they are not used in the same way.

- **Baker's yeast:** Baker's yeast is purchased alive and used to leaven bread and other baked goods. The yeast is killed during cooking but adds an earthy, yeasty flavor when used in baking. It is a source of proteins, B vitamins, and minerals, although once baked, the nutritional values are diminished.
- **Brewer's yeast:** Brewer's yeast can be purchased alive and is used to brew beer. The dead yeast cells leftover from the brewing process are also sold to be be consumed as a nutritional supplement in the form of powder, flakes, and tablets. You can add nutritional Brewer's yeast to smoothies, cereals, salads, soups, and stews, and it is a rich source of B vitamins and minerals, including chromium, selenium, zinc, and iron. The flavor is distinctive and bitter and not to everyone's taste.

- **Nutritional yeast:** This yeast is grown specifically to be used as a food product. The yeast cells are killed during manufacturing and not alive in the final product. It is used in cooking and has a cheesy, nutty, or savory flavor.
- **Yeast extract:** A concentrated, savory flavoring made from yeast. It is commonly used in the food industry to enhance the taste of various products. The process of making yeast extract involves breaking down yeast cells to release their contents, which include proteins, vitamins, and other flavor compounds. Well-known brand names for yeast extracts are Marmite in the UK and Vegemite in Australia.

Marmite vs. Vegemite

MARMITE
Ingredients: Yeast extract, salt, vegetable juice concentrate, riboflavin, niacin, thiamine, vitamin B12, folic acid, and spices.

Flavor: Marmite has a savory, salty, and slightly bitter flavor. Some people describe it as having a richer taste compared to Vegemite.

VEGEMITE
Ingredients: Saccharomyces cerevisiae yeast extract, salt, malt extract, color additive (caramel to give it the dark color), thiamine, riboflavin, niacin, and folate, and vegetable juice concentrate.

Flavor: Vegemite has a salty, umami-rich flavor. It is known for its savory and slightly bitter taste. Some people find Vegemite to be milder than Marmite.

WHAT IS AQUAFABA?

Aquafaba is a word made from an amalgamation of the Latin words for water and bean and is a vegan ingredient that is often used to replace eggs when cooking. You can easily make it at home using the leftover juice from a can of legumes such as chickpeas.

Aquafaba is the "juice" of legumes that have been soaked or cooked in water for long periods of time. Usually chickpeas are used to create it as they produce the most starchy liquid and a neutral flavor. Legume seeds like chickpeas and soybeans contain some of the same proteins found in eggs, which is partly why they can be used to create foam in the same way. A study has found that the main components of aquafaba are polysaccharides, sucrose, and various proteins, which contain the same chemical components as egg white. The saponins that are formed when the aquafaba is shaken creates a foam similar to egg whites.

Eggs act as coagulators in recipes, and they are more difficult to replace than some other animal products if you are consuming a vegan diet. Eggs

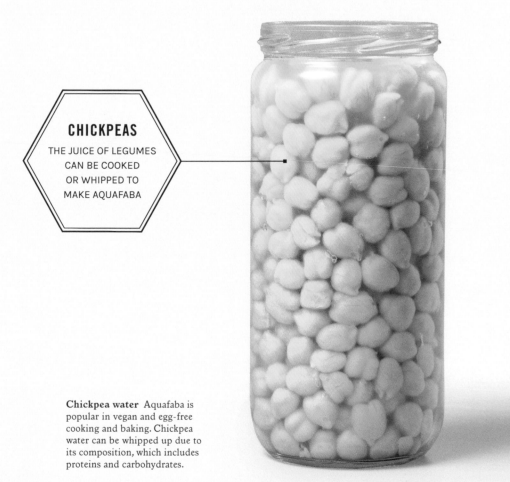

CHICKPEAS
THE JUICE OF LEGUMES CAN BE COOKED OR WHIPPED TO MAKE AQUAFABA

Chickpea water Aquafaba is popular in vegan and egg-free cooking and baking. Chickpea water can be whipped up due to its composition, which includes proteins and carbohydrates.

HOW MUCH SHOULD I USE?

HERE'S HOW MUCH AQUAFABA YOU NEED TO REPLACE EGGS:

1 EGG YOLK
1 tbsp aquafaba

1 EGG WHITE
2 tbsp aquafaba

1 WHOLE EGG
3 tbsp aquafaba

change to a solid state when either heat, strong acids, or an alkaline cause the proteins in them to denature (break down their structure). The speed and quality of this process depends on the salt, sugar, and acid content of the food. The key proteins in eggs are conalbumin and ovalbumin in the white and lipoproteins in the yolk (see pp.54–55). While you can recreate some of the texture of eggs using aquafaba in recipes, you cannot replicate their nutritional qualities. Aquafaba on its own has no significant nutritional value.

HOW IS AQUAFABA MADE?

You can buy aquafaba, but it is probably easier and cheaper to make your own. The quickest method is to use a can of chickpeas that are low in salt, shake the can, and drain the liquid to use in your cooking. You can make aquafaba by soaking and cooking dried chickpeas, draining the chickpeas, and then simmering the juice until it reaches the consistency of egg white. This method takes a lot longer. If you are using it as a replacement for egg white, you'll need to whisk it for up to 10 minutes.

HOW TO USE AQUAFABA

Aquafaba can be used in place of egg white in baking and can also be added to soups or vegan butters or to make a creamy hummus. You may need to experiment to get the right amount of aquafaba. Try aquafaba as an egg replacement in the following:

- Meringue or pavlova
- Pancakes
- Muffins
- Chocolate mousse
- Vegan ice cream
- Mayonnaise
- Vegan butter

For mayonnaise, take 3 tbsp aquafaba, 2 tsp Dijon mustard, ¾ tsp salt, ¼ tsp fine white pepper, 2 tbsp white wine vinegar, and 1 cup (250ml) of a neutral oil, such as vegetable oil. Whisk together the ingredients and use as you would mayonnaise.

To make chocolate mousse, melt 7oz (200g) of dark chocolate and let cool. Whisk ½ cup (120ml) of aquafaba and ½ cup (100g) of powdered sugar until stiff peaks are formed. Add in the cooled melted chocolate and mix in. Spoon the mixture into serving bowls and chill for an hour minimum.

What are saponins?

COMPOUNDS CALLED SAPONINS ARE WITHIN THE CELLS OF ALL LEGUME PLANTS SUCH AS CHICKPEAS.

These compounds get their name from the Latin word "sapo," meaning soap. This is due to their ability to form stable, soaplike foams in aqueous solutions and is one of the reasons aquafaba can be used in some recipes to replace egg whites. Saponins have antioxidant properties and help modulate the immune system. They can also help reduce cholesterol absorption in the body. However, saponins can act as antinutrients by binding to minerals, including zinc, calcium, and iron, which may lead to nutrient deficiencies. Some people may be allergic to saponins. In very high doses, saponins are toxic, although this is unlikely to affect you and will not happen if eaten as part of a normal dietary intake.

SHOULD I EAT NUT BUTTERS?

Nut butters can be a very helpful way of including additional beneficial fats and nutrients into your diet, but the quality and quantity of the nut butters consumed matter.

———————

Nut butters are nuts that have been ground down and made into a paste, which can then be spread like butter. Any nut can be made into a nut butter from popular well-known varieties of peanut butters, almonds butters, and cashew butters to less-known options of pistachio, macadamia, and pecan butters. Not all nut butters are just nuts; when choosing the nut butter, always check the ingredients as some varieties have added palm oil, sugars, and salts and best avoided—opt for 100 percent nuts. Consuming nuts in the right amounts has been shown to support weight loss and reduce your risk of diabetes, heart disease, and some cancers. They also provide an array of healthy fats, fiber, polyphenols, and vitamins.

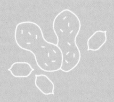

Nut butter comparisons

Nut butters are an easy way to to include some nuts in your weekly diet. A handful of a variety of nuts eaten a few times a week will be enough to benefit from their healthy fats, protein, fiber, and minerals.

PEANUT BUTTER

Higher in protein than almond butter. Contains iron, potassium, magnesium, vitamin B6, and zinc. One of the most studied nut butters, research suggests that consuming this regularly is good for heart health and those with diabetes.

ALMOND BUTTER

Highest in healthy fats, 3g more of heart-healthy monounsaturated fat per serving compared to peanut butter. (It's also slightly higher in nutrients like the antioxidant vitamin E.) Almond butter can be more expensive than peanut butter.

PER SERVING (2 TBSP)	PER SERVING (2 TBSP)
191 CALORIES	196 CALORIES
16.4g FAT	17.8g FAT
7.1g CARBS	6g CARBS
1.6g FIBER	3.3g FIBER
3.4g SUGAR	2g SUGAR
136mg SALT	73mg SALT
7.1g PROTEIN	7g PROTEIN

Try adding nut butters to your breakfast cereals, oatmeal, yogurt, smoothies, or curries, or make frozen fruit and nut butter slices. Nut butter is a good addition to a snack—such as apple and peanut butter—as it can help stabilize blood sugar levels.

TOO MUCH FAT?

Some people are reluctant to eat nut butters because there is a perception that they have a high fat content. However, these are essential, healthy fats, and not saturated. The amount

PROTEIN PACKED

NUTS CONTAIN AROUND 20g OF PROTEIN PER 100g. A SERVING IS 2 TBSP (32g).

of fat absorbed varies widely between different people. Also, it is believed that not all the fat contained in nuts is absorbed by the body, due to their fibrous cell wall structure. Some of the fat makes its way through your digestive system and is released at the other end. The amount you absorb can also be affected by the way the nuts are prepared. Chopping, chewing, and blending breaks down their cellular structure and releases more fat. Generally, you shouldn't avoid nuts unless you have an allergy as they contain many healthy nutrients.

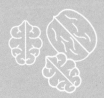

HAZELNUT BUTTER

Contains oleic acid, a form of monounsaturated fat that may help lower your risk of heart disease and stroke. A source of vitamin E and a good option if allergic to peanuts.

PER SERVING (2 TBSP)

160 CALORIES

14g FAT

8g CARBS

1g FIBER

0g SUGAR

0mg SALT

5g PROTEIN

CASHEW BUTTER

Naturally sweet and with less protein than some other nut butters, cashew butter does contain some iron and B vitamins.

PER SERVING (2 TBSP)

195 CALORIES

17g FAT

9.7g CARBS

1g FIBER

3g SUGAR

94mg SALT

3.9g PROTEIN

WALNUT BUTTER

Contains alpha-linoleic acid (ALA), the omega-3 found in plants, which helps lower the risk of heart disease. Also contains monounsaturated fats and vitamin E.

PER SERVING (2 TBSP)

170 CALORIES

14g FAT

11g CARBS

1g FIBER

7g SUGAR

0mg SALT

3g PROTEIN

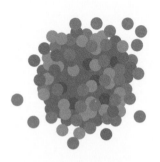

Lentils

A good source of protein, fiber, and iron. Add lentils to soups, stews, and salads. Make lentil burgers or lentil shepherd's pie.

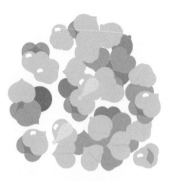

Chickpeas

A good source of folate, manganese, and phosphorus. Use in hummus or roast them and add to salads for texture and extra protein.

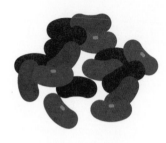

Kidney beans

A good source of protein, fiber, iron, potassium, magnesium, and vitamin K. Use in burrito bowls, tacos, and chili.

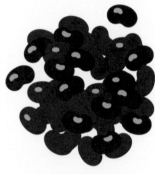

Black beans

A rich source of antioxidants, including anthocyanins. Make black bean soup, burgers, or burritos.

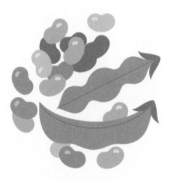

Soybeans

A source of omega-3 fatty acids, isoflavones, and saponins. Use soybean tofu in stir-fries and add to soup. Use tempeh in sandwiches.

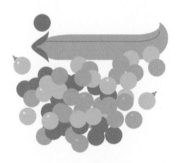

Green peas

Nutritious and balanced as a source of carbs, protein, fiber, vitamins C, A, and K. Add to salads, soups, and stews.

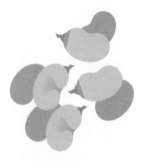

Broad beans

Whether fresh or dried as fava beans, they're a good source of vitamins B1, B2, and B6. Use in soups, add to risotto or pasta dishes, or use as a meat substitute.

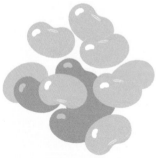

Lima beans

Rich in vitamins A, C, and K. Use in soups or eat them roasted. They make a creamy dip.

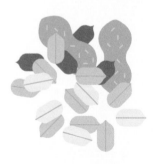

Peanuts

High in heart-healthy fats and vitamins E and B. Use in a peanut sauce in stir-fries, or eat them as they are.

SHOULD I EAT MORE BEANS, PEAS, AND LENTILS?

Beans, peas, chickpeas, and lentils are a great way to add flavor and nutrition to plant dishes. They are affordable and beneficial for your health, and you should aim to eat a variety of them through the week.

There are many types of beans and lentils that you can include in your plant-based diet, and they have important benefits for health. This group of foods are sometimes also referred to as legumes or pulses. Legumes are plants that produce seeds in pods and include beans, lentils, peas, chickpeas, soybeans, and peanuts. Pulses are part of the legume family, but pulses are dried before they are eaten (so fresh peas are legumes; dried peas are pulses).

HEALTH BENEFITS

Legumes and pulses are high in protein and fiber and low in fat, making them the perfect addition to everyone's diet. A lot of research suggests that eating legumes and pulses roughly four times a week can cut your risk of coronary disease by 14 percent. Other studies have shown that eating these foods four times a week may lead to a 22 percent lower risk of heart disease and an 11 percent lower risk of cardiovascular disease, compared to those who eat them less than once a week.

Their health-giving properties may be due to the fiber, folate, and phytochemicals (see pp.68–69) they contain. The fiber in legumes especially may help lower blood cholesterol even without weight loss, and may prevent sharp rises in blood sugar, both of which are risk factors for type 2 diabetes and cardiovascular disease.

Their mix of protein and fiber keeps you fuller for longer as they are digested slowly. One portion of legumes or pulses (three heaped tablespoons) provides up to 9g of protein—about a sixth of what you need in a day. One can of kidney beans contains as much protein as a portion of ground beef and almost no fat or salt (check the label for added salt).

Eating legumes is also cost-effective, because they are a much cheaper source of protein compared with animal products.

THE ENVIRONMENTAL IMPACT

The environment will also benefit by all of us eating more legumes and pulses because they don't need much water or fertilizer, and they even improve the soil for other crops. They are able to convert nitrogen in the atmosphere into a form that can be used by plants for growth. Legumes generally have a lower carbon footprint than other forms of protein as their cultivation uses less energy and emits fewer greenhouse gases than meat production.

THE BEST WAY TO EAT BEANS, PEAS, AND LENTILS

A great way to consume legumes is to buy canned beans and lentils—you can use them straight from the can (choose the ones without added salt) and then add them to a variety of recipes. You can also buy pulses and cook them efficiently using a pressure cooker (see pp.156–157). In this way, you can easily bulk up your regular recipes, for example, by adding kidney beans to your favorite chili. Hummus is a great dip to make using chickpeas, and you can add extra pulses to your favorite soups and salads at lunch. To help you make a switch from meat, start with half and half. One way to do this is to make a bolognese with half lentils and half meat (see p.50).

WHAT ARE THE BEST GRAINS TO EAT?

Grains are a type of carbohydrate you should aspire to consume as part of a healthy balanced diet, as they contain fiber and beneficial vitamins and minerals. Grains are the seeds of crops such as barley, oats, rice, and wheat.

WHOLE GRAINS

When it comes to grains, the advice is to stick to whole grains where possible. Grains are considered whole grain when the bran and germ of the grain is not removed during processing and refining. The bran and germ contain important nutrients that have benefits for our health. There is a breadth of evidence to support this advice. Analysis published in the *Lancet* took 185 prospective studies and 58 clinical trials combined to assess the markers of human health associated with carbohydrate quality. Higher consumers of whole grains demonstrated a significantly lower risk of all-cause mortality (–19 percent), coronary heart disease (–20 percent), type 2 diabetes (–33 percent), and cancer mortality (–16 percent) compared with lower consumers. Similar results were found for fiber intake, indicating this may be the beneficial nutrient in whole grains.

PSEUDOGRAINS

So-called "pseudograins," including quinoa, buckwheat, and amaranth, aren't technically grains; they are the seeds of broadleaf plants. However, they behave similarly and so are used in the same ways. These are often eaten in their unrefined forms although sometimes their outer husks are removed, which can affect their nutrient content. One of the great things about pseudograins is that they're naturally gluten-free, so they suit a wide variety of dietary needs. Compared to wheat, pseudograins are a richer source of complete protein, fiber, iron, and magnesium, and many provide far more calcium. Eating them can improve low intakes of these micronutrients in plant-based diets and help combat losses from antinutrient activity because pseudograins are lower in antinutrients (see p.91) than some traditional grains.

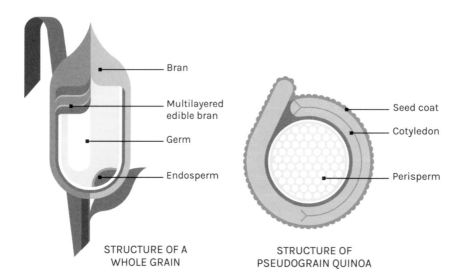

Bran

Multilayered edible bran

Germ

Endosperm

STRUCTURE OF A WHOLE GRAIN

Seed coat

Cotyledon

Perisperm

STRUCTURE OF PSEUDOGRAIN QUINOA

Whole grains and unrefined pseudograins Look for versions that are in their whole form and so have higher nutritional benefits than refined versions.

Whole grains Some examples of whole grains to include in your diet are shown here. Eating a great variety is beneficial for gut health.

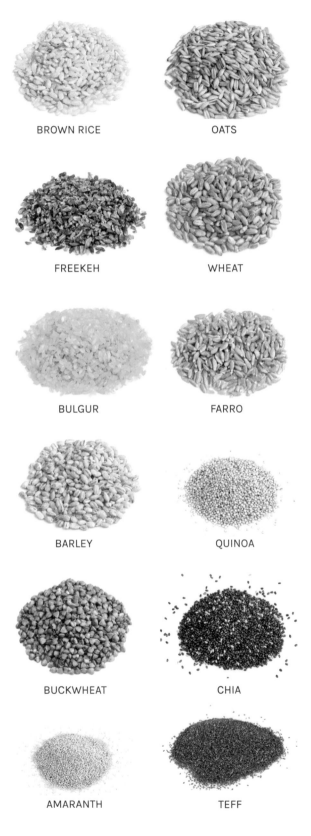

BROWN RICE

OATS

FREEKEH

WHEAT

BULGUR

FARRO

BARLEY

QUINOA

BUCKWHEAT

CHIA

AMARANTH

TEFF

REFINED GRAINS

Refined grains differ from whole grains as they have the fiber-rich bran and micronutrient-rich germ removed during processing, leaving the starch-rich endosperm. Many refined grains are fortified with micronutrients, such as B vitamins and iron, to compensate for the loss of naturally occurring nutrients in the germ. Refined grains don't appear to have the same nutritional and health benefits as whole grains. They may also not be as filling and satisfying as whole grains due to their reduced fiber content, which might be a contributing factor to the results of research indicating refined grains are linked with higher body weight. It isn't the grain itself that causes weight gain but rather the increased calorie intake caused by eating a larger quantity to feel satisfied. Refined grain foods generally appear to be digested more quickly and raise blood glucose levels faster than whole grains.

However, evidence for refined grains being "bad" for health is inconclusive—the only compelling research seems to be that increased consumption of certain refined grains, like white rice, seem to be linked with increased risk of negative health outcomes such as type 2 diabetes in certain populations, particularly in India, China, and other parts of Asia where consumption regularly exceeds recommendations. It may be the case that whole grains are "good," but refined grains aren't "bad." Ultimately, we know variety is key to a healthy gut, which in turn is linked to a whole host of health benefits. There's no single grain we should stick to eating for optimal health and nutritional benefits, but instead incorporating a mixture of different grains helps us harness the pros of each.

WHICH DAIRY-FREE PRODUCTS SHOULD I CHOOSE?

Dairy foods are made from animal milk. You may choose to reduce your intake of these products or cut them out of your diet altogether for ethical and environmental reasons. With so many alternative products available, which should you buy?

REASONS FOR GOING DAIRY-FREE

There are many reasons people choose to stop consuming dairy foods. It may be a personal choice for ethical or environmental reasons. Often, it is due to allergies or intolerances, which mean people cannot eat products that contain dairy or cow's milk. It's also important to know that dairy-free products may not suit everyone due to some of the ingredients that are added, so check the labels.

Dairy milk and its alternatives

While dairy milk contains many healthy nutrients naturally, you can find plant-based alternatives with vitamins and minerals added. Here is a comparison of nutrients per 100ml of cow's milk and plant milks.

Over the years a huge array of dairy-free and lactose-free alternatives to cow's milk have been introduced to the market. These include soy, rice, oat, nut, pea, quinoa, and even potato milks, as well as cheeses, yogurts, cream and ice cream, and butter fats made from plant-based produce. With such a huge choice available, it can be difficult to know which ones to try. It may come down to your taste, but you also need to think about the nutritional values of the products available.

NUTRIENTS

Compared to dairy, plant-based dairy-free products contain less calcium, phosphorus, magnesium, potassium, and sodium and fewer vitamins such as vitamins D and B12. A recent study of nearly 300 plant-based dairy alternatives found that only 57 percent of milk alternatives, 63 percent of yogurt alternatives, and 28 percent of cheese alternatives are

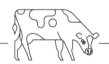

COW'S MILK

A good source of calcium and proteins but higher carbon footprint than plant milks.

ENERGY 47KCAL
FAT 1.8g
PROTEIN 3.6g
CALCIUM 120mg

ALMOND MILK

Low in protein and fat. Contains natural vitamin E, good for skin and eyes.

ENERGY 13KCAL
FAT 1.1g
PROTEIN 0.5g
CALCIUM 120mg

SOY MILK

A good alternative as soybeans are a rich source of protein.

ENERGY 33KCAL
FAT 1.8g
PROTEIN 3.3g
CALCIUM 120mg

OAT MILK

Contains fiber, which can help lower cholesterol. Oats use less water to grow than cow's milk.

ENERGY 46KCAL
FAT 1.5g
PROTEIN 1g
CALCIUM 120mg

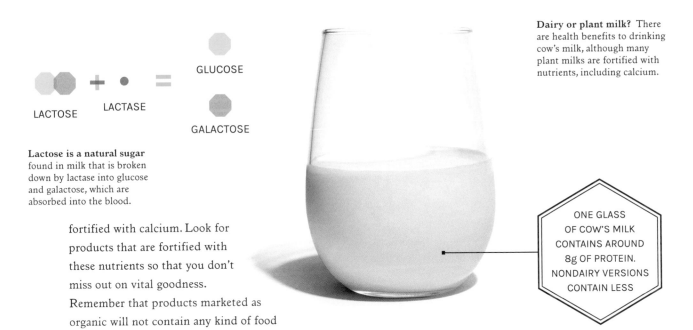

GLUCOSE

LACTOSE   LACTASE

GALACTOSE

Lactose is a natural sugar found in milk that is broken down by lactase into glucose and galactose, which are absorbed into the blood.

Dairy or plant milk? There are health benefits to drinking cow's milk, although many plant milks are fortified with nutrients, including calcium.

ONE GLASS OF COW'S MILK CONTAINS AROUND 8g OF PROTEIN. NONDAIRY VERSIONS CONTAIN LESS

fortified with calcium. Look for products that are fortified with these nutrients so that you don't miss out on vital goodness. Remember that products marketed as organic will not contain any kind of food fortification due to the methods of processing. Also, check dairy-free products for artificial sweeteners and added sugars. Most of us are already consuming too much sugar, so it's best to choose unsweetened versions of dairy-free foods.

LACTOSE-FREE OR DAIRY-FREE?

When products are lactose-free, they do not contain the sugar called lactose that is found in milk, but they do still contain dairy. Dairy-free products, on the other hand, do not contain any dairy at all. Lactase is the body's own enzyme that breaks down lactose into glucose and galactose so they can be absorbed through the intestinal wall and into our bloodstream. Those with a lactose allergy or intolerance, where the enzyme lactase is not present or doesn't function as effectively, may feel discomfort as lactose isn't broken down into galactose and glucose in the intestines. There are now multiple options out there for those with lactose intolerances or allergies to choose from that still allow them to enjoy the taste of dairy.

CASHEW NUT

Contains low levels of fat and protein, largely made of water with 3% cashews.

ENERGY 23KCAL
FAT 1.1g
PROTEIN 0.5g
CALCIUM 120mg

COCONUT MILK

Similar fat levels to cow's milk, although coconut farming has led to deforestation.

ENERGY 15KCAL
FAT 1.3g
PROTEIN 0.7g
CALCIUM 120mg

RICE MILK

Rice production causes high carbon emissions. Contains more calories than some milks.

ENERGY 50KCAL
FAT 1g
PROTEIN 0.1g
CALCIUM 120mg

HAZELNUT MILK

Low in calories and fat, and the cultivation of hazelnuts is less harmful than some other nuts.

ENERGY 29KCAL
FAT 1.6g
PROTEIN 0.4g
CALCIUM 120mg

SHOULD WE BE EATING ALGAE?

Humans have eaten macroalgae (seaweed) and microalgae (aquatic microorganisms) for thousands of years. They can be a useful part of a plant-based diet because they are rich in protein, amino acids, fatty acids, and vitamins. Popular examples are wakame, spirulina, chlorella, and nori seaweed.

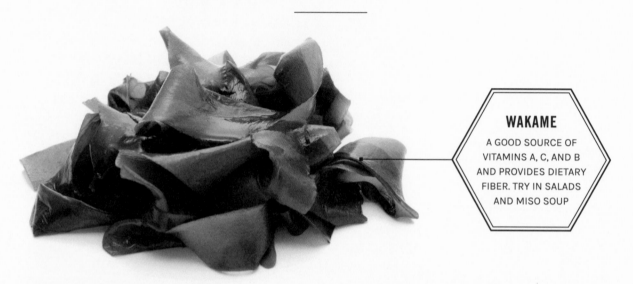

WAKAME

A GOOD SOURCE OF VITAMINS A, C, AND B AND PROVIDES DIETARY FIBER. TRY IN SALADS AND MISO SOUP

Algae are protein-rich organisms found in fresh and seawater. They are either harvested from the wild or grown for human consumption and eaten fresh, dried, or pickled. They can be very nutrient-rich, but this depends on the type of algae consumed. Some contain essential amino acids; essential fatty acids, including omega-3, omega-6, and omega-7; along with vitamins such as A, D, and E. While there is some evidence for microalgae being beneficial to human health, further scientific research is needed to fully understand its impacts, effects, and benefits. Seaweed, spirulina, and chlorella are all nutritious whole foods that are sources of essential nutrients.

THE BENEFITS OF SPIRULINA

Spirulina is rich in protein, thiamine, riboflavin, niacin, copper, and iron. Spirulina consumption has been linked to lower low-density lipoprotein (LDL) or

"bad" cholesterol and lower fat levels in the blood, lower blood pressure, and blood sugar improvement. Further research has shown that eating spirulina can help our immune systems and cause an increase of hemoglobin levels of red blood cells in older people. Hemoglobin is a protein in red blood cells that carries oxygen from the lungs to the rest of the body. Having an increase in hemoglobin levels will improve oxygen transport around the body.

CHLORELLA

Chlorella (also known as *Chlorella vulgaris*) is a fresh water microalgae that is usually taken as a supplement in a tablet or powder form that can be added to sweet or savory recipes. It contains an abundance of antioxidants, such as vitamin C, lutein, carotenoids, and tocopherol; as well as protein; fat; minerals; and other vitamins, such as vitamins B1,

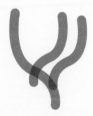

MACROALGAE

Macroalgaes, including edible seaweed such as nori, wakame, dulse, and kombu, are often consumed as snacks or in a variety of dishes.

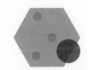

MICROALGAE

Microalgaes like spirulina and chlorella are available in powdered form and can be eaten sprinkled over food or blended into juices and smoothies.

B2, B6, B12, D2, E, and K. It also contains substantial amounts of iron (104mg/100g dry weight) and potassium (986mg/100g dry weight) and selenium. Studies suggest that chlorella can improve cholesterol levels, blood pressure, and blood glucose levels after overnight fasting (8–12 hours while sleeping).

WAKAME

Wakame is an edible seaweed that has been eaten in Japan and Korea for centuries and is also now grown along the west coast of North America, Europe, New Zealand, and Australia. Wakame is linked to lower cholesterol levels and decreased blood pressure and is a good source of iodine. It may contain high levels of sodium and salt and some heavy metals such as arsenic depending on the water contamination from where wakame is grown. Eaten in moderation (less than about 10g a day), this does not present a risk to health.

NORI

Nori is an edible red algae that grows on rocks in shallow seas. Possibly the most well-known type of edible seaweed, nori was originally used in Japanese cuisine as dried sheets (thin sushi rolls). Research suggests compounds obtained through eating nori may help with our overall gut health, lower LDL-cholesterol, and have anti-tumor properties.

Microalgae cultivation

MICROALGAE IS GROWN FOR HUMAN CONSUMPTION IN CONTROLLED ENVIRONMENTS THAT ARE DESIGNED FOR OPTIMUM GROWTH.

SPECIES SELECTION

THERE ARE DIFFERENT SPECIES OF MICROALGAE THAT CAN BE GROWN DEPENDING ON THEIR END USE

OPEN POND OR BIOREACTOR

LARGE SHALLOW PONDS ARE FILLED WITH ALGAE CULTURE, OR CLOSED BIOREACTORS CAN BE USED. NUTRIENTS FOR GROWTH ARE SUPPLIED

LIGHT AND TEMPERATURE

NATURAL OR ARTIFICIAL LIGHT IS PROVIDED SO THE ALGAE CAN PHOTOSYNTHESIZE AND TEMPERATURE IS CONTROLLED TO GAIN MAXIMUM YIELD AND QUALITY

HARVESTING

COLLECTION TAKES PLACE ONCE THE ALGAE HAVE REACHED THE DESIRED SIZE. THEN IT MAY BE AIR-DRIED, FREEZE-DRIED, OR SPRAY-DRIED

PROCESSING

THE DRIED ALGAE CAN BE MADE INTO FOODS OR SUPPLEMENTS, OR USED IN OTHER PRODUCTS LIKE FUEL

WHAT IS CULTURED MEAT?

Scientists are able to grow animal cells in a sterile laboratory environment, which can be used to produce lab-grown or cultured meat. This could be a promising addition in the food chain to support the environment, but is it wholly ethical?

———

Cultured meat, also known as lab-grown meat or clean meat, is made from the same animal tissue as natural meat. However, instead of being grown inside an animal's body, it is grown in a laboratory. This is done by removing a small number of muscle cells from a living animal. It is possible to take these cells from the animal typically using local anesthesia to provide relief from pain. The animal may experience a momentary twinge of discomfort, not unlike the feeling of getting a routine blood test at the doctor's, according to scientists. The cells are placed into bioreactors and then transferred to a bath of nutrients where they grow into muscle tissue, which scientists transform using edible scaffolding. This is a way of holding together muscle fat and connective tissue that resembles the structure of naturally produced meat. This tissue

can be manipulated into chicken nuggets, burgers, or steaks. At the moment, cultured meat is not widely available, but companies around the world are currently working on ways to produce lab-grown lamb, beef, chicken, and seafood. It could be available to buy in restaurants and supermarkets and become part of our diets in the near future.

WHAT ARE THE BENEFITS?

● **Environmental:** The UN cites livestock production as a "key factor" in deforestation and approximately 30 percent of the Earth's land mass is used to graze animals or grow feed crops for them. In terms of greenhouse gas emissions, the production and consumption of cultured meat may be a better long-term choice than more traditional farming methods as it relies on fewer livestock, although more

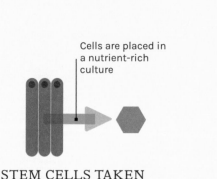

Cells are placed in a nutrient-rich culture

STEM CELLS TAKEN

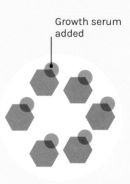

Growth serum added

CELLS MULTIPLY

Cultured meat production

Meat can now be grown in a lab using stem cells from an animal. It is not considered vegan because the end product is the same as traditionally created meat.

Muscle stem cells are retrieved from a living animal or from existing cell banks. This is a relatively painless procedure for the animal. Stem cells are used because they can be turned into any product.

Growth serums are added to cells, which are nurtured in a petri dish so they multiply.

studies are needed to confirm this. Artificial or lab-grown meat also does not lead to massive carbon dioxide and methane emissions that damage the climate: scientists estimate that industrialized cultured meat production would generate 78–96 percent less greenhouse gas than conventional factory farming.

- **Feeding the world:** Cultured meat could help us feed the hungry in a time of food insecurity. Eating meat is hugely inefficient because of all the grain consumed by farmed animals, which could instead be eaten by humans. Cells taken from a single cow can produce an astonishing 175 million quarter-pounder burgers made from cultured meat.
- **A safer option:** Meat produced in a laboratory is also safer for human consumption. The sterile environment eliminates infections with bacteria such as E. coli, campylobacter, and salmonella from factory-farm germs. Cultured meat is also free of the antibiotics that permeate a lot of farmed animal products.
- **Ethical:** Cultured meat is not cruel, it does not harm animals, and it reduces the need for slaughterhouses.

- **Nutrition:** Nutritionally speaking, it is still early days in the production of cultured meat, but the protein produced would match that of the meat produced from killing an animal. Due to its high cholesterol and saturated fat content, we know that meat consumption can increase risk of disease. But when growing meat in a lab, food scientists can control the quantities of harmful cholesterol and saturated fat it contains, making it a healthier alternative.

SHOULD I EAT IT?

There are a few reasons why people may not wish to eat meat created in a lab. For those concerned with animal welfare, some animals will still be needed for this process. Other objections may be religious and cultural, while some may not want to eat something that is seen as unnatural. Further, it is not yet clear how the control of nutrients in the meat will be regulated, particularly in terms of micronutrients and iron. Finally, it is also likely that some people will still prefer to avoid eating meat, even if it is created without harming any living animals.

PRODUCTION OF 1kg OF BEEF PRODUCES

300kg CO_2 equivalent

uses **15,000** litres of water

needs **400m²** land

70% MORE FOOD WILL BE NEEDED BY 2050 TO MEET THE NEEDS OF A GROWING GLOBAL POPULATION

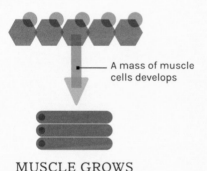

MUSCLE GROWS

A mass of muscle cells develops

As the cells multiply, they create muscle tissue, which is what is normally eaten in traditional meat.

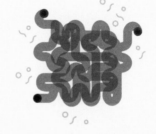

MEAT PROCESSING

The muscle cells are put into a bioreactor and grown into strands that resemble meat. Flavorings and nutrients are added.

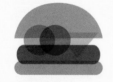

CONSUMPTION

The strands are used to create a meat product. For example, 20,000 strands will make one hamburger.

IS 3D FOOD PRINTING THE FUTURE?

Scientists are working hard to find more sustainable ways to feed an ever-increasing population. 3D printing is a new and novel technology that could revolutionize the way we produce food.

———————

The global meat industry produced 82.7 million tons (75 million metric tons) of meat in 2020, around 19lb (8.6kg) for each person on the planet. There is a huge and growing demand for meat worldwide, and scientists are working to meet this demand with alternatives to traditionally produced animal products. The alternative meat industry is worth approximately 5.6 billion dollars.

HOW DOES 3D PRINTING PRODUCE FOOD?

3D food printing is one option scientists are exploring. To create meat products without the need for livestock farming, animal cells called starter cells are isolated and grown in a bioreactor to produce a large quantity of biomass (see pp.138–139). The cells are divided into two categories of edible tissue—muscle cells and fat cells—which are then printed into meat. Some consider this meat to be vegetarian or vegan as there is no ethical violation in eating printed meat made using cultured animal cells, although others may disagree. The printed meat is then fed into a 3D printer. Imagine a normal household printer with ink, but you feed it material you can eat. The end product is then cooked.

HOW IS IT BEING USED?

Currently in order to 3D print food, you require a pastelike consistency from foods like purées, mousses, and chocolate ganache. However, there still appears to be technical challenges that need to be addressed to help increase the availability and acceptability of 3D foods to the general public. Many of the 3D foods currently available involve the following ingredients:

- Purée
- Jelly

THE 3D FOOD PRINTING PROCESS

1.
POWDER BED
The process begins with a thin layer of material spread evenly over a build platform. The material used in this case may be an edible resin.

2.
LASER SCANNING
A high-powered laser is used to selectively scan and heat the edible material to make it more malleable and prepare it for printing.

3.
LAYER-BY-LAYER
The food is created one layer at a time. The edible resin is pushed through a dispenser called an extruder and gradually built up as the printer follows a preprogrammed recipe.

- Cheese
- Chocolate
- Sauces
- Icing
- Mashed potatoes
- Protein powder
- Sugar
- Colored food ink

CHOCOLATE

ONE OF THE PRODUCTS THAT CAN BE CREATED USING 3D PRINTING METHODS

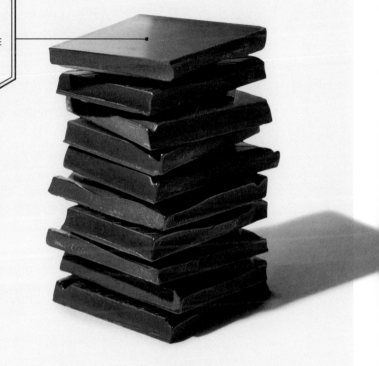

WHAT ABOUT MEAT SUBSTITUTES?

Some versions of different meat substitutes are in development. Companies are currently using 3D printing to produce meat substitutes made from plants. Some of the ingredients include pea protein and beet juice to make a plant-based steak product. Others are working on printing 3D pizzas, which can be used to feed travelers in space. Approval from the Food and Drug Administration that deemed one particular brand's lab-grown cultivated chicken safe to eat also gained approval from the US Department of Agriculture. This means that their products may be sold, although we cannot yet buy them widely.

WHAT ARE THE BENEFITS?

If 3D printing of meat becomes more widespread, it would bring many benefits. It may help reduce world hunger by providing a much-needed new source of food. It would produce 90 percent less greenhouse gas emissions than livestock farming, which causes deforestation and increasing levels of CO_2, and so it would benefit the environment. Importantly, 3D meat can be made without the need to slaughter animals or cause any cruelty and so may appeal to some plant-based eaters. This technology could also be used to improve the nutrition of people around the world as the protein, vitamin, and mineral levels it contains can be carefully controlled. In the future, you may even be able to tailor the levels of nutrients in your food to suit your individual needs.

At the moment, there is limited research on this new technology analyzing its impact on both human health and the environment. 3D is still in the early days of innovation and has some way to go before we see it used by professionals and consumers;however, it is an area to keep an eye on.

4.
COOLING AND SOLIDIFICATION

Once the food is dispensed, the material cools and solidifies, forming a three-dimensional food product.

5.
SUPPORT STRUCTURES

In some cases, support structures made of the same material as the food itself may be added during the printing process. These are removed later.

SHOULD I PAY ATTENTION TO FOOD LABELS?

It is important to have a rough understanding of what ingredients go into the products we buy as this can have an impact on our overall health. Added ingredients are sometimes important and at other times are included purely for taste.

To make a healthy choice in a plant-based market, it is important to understand labels. It has been proven that healthier choices are often made when food labels are read, but understanding what's on those labels isn't always straightforward.

FORTIFICATION

As a plant-based eater, it is important to understand how to check for fortification (added minerals and vitamins) because you may not be getting all the nutrients needed to stay healthy by eating plant foods alone (see pp.96–97). Usually, if a plant-based food is fortified, this is a benefit to the product as it will include more nutrients. However, not all plant-based foods are fortified and not all contain the right fortifications. Some data suggests, for example, that only 45 percent of yogurts are fortified with

calcium to at least 5 percent of the daily recommendation and only one-fifth are fortified with vitamins B12 and D, which are vital to the health of plant-based eaters in particular.

Well-planned vegetarian and vegan diets can provide most essential nutrients, but there are some that may be more difficult to get enough of (such as vitamin B12), or which might be less absorbed by the body from plant-based foods (such as iron, zinc, and calcium). Fortified foods (fortified breakfast cereals or plant milks) may be useful for providing these nutrients.

It's also important to read food labels to check for high levels of sugar, salt, and fats, which can lead to health issues. According to the World Health Organization, programs for fortification need to work alongside policies designed to reduce disease.

Monitor your sugar, fat, and salt

Sugar, saturated fat, and salt intake should be controlled as part of healthy eating. Use these steps to become more aware of how much you eat in each meal or snack and over a whole day.

   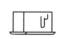

Know the daily limits These are the recommended daily intake amounts from the Dietary Guidelines for Americans.	CALORIES	ADDED SUGAR	TOTAL FAT	SATURATED FAT	SALT
	2,000	**<25g**	**<78g**	**<22g**	**<2,300mg**

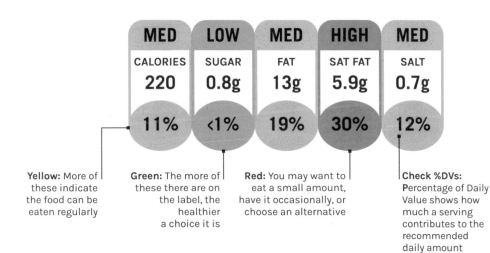

MED	LOW	MED	HIGH	MED
CALORIES	SUGAR	FAT	SAT FAT	SALT
220	0.8g	13g	5.9g	0.7g
11%	<1%	19%	30%	12%

Yellow: More of these indicate the food can be eaten regularly

Green: The more of these there are on the label, the healthier a choice it is

Red: You may want to eat a small amount, have it occasionally, or choose an alternative

Check %DVs: Percentage of Daily Value shows how much a serving contributes to the recommended daily amount

Food labels Many countries have adopted similar labeling systems so that you can quickly see whether the food you're buying is high or low in calories, sugar, salt, and fat.

For example, salt iodization, which helps increase intake of iodine, has the negative effect of increasing salt consumption. Another example is yogurts, half of which have been found to have high levels of sugar, while the coconut plant-based alternatives were higher in saturated fat than the dairy alternatives.

LABEL PSYCHOLOGY

Interestingly, when asking consumers what they looked for on food labels, there was a direct gender divide with more women than men looking at the nutritional information, and a large majority looking at the food itself to make a judgment on its taste, rather than reading the labels. More consumers who read the labels worry about the additives, country of origin, and ingredient quality than the nutritional quality, and studies suggest the language on the product itself is a dictating factor of consumption. One study found that meat-based products

used language that induced consumers to want to eat, whereas plant-based products didn't. When plant-based products did use this language, meat-eaters were more inclined to want to eat that product. This suggests that if we want to increase plant eating, we need to change the way products are labeled.

READING FOOD LABELS

Often consumers look only at the front of a food package rather than the more detailed nutrition label on the back, which is why some countries have developed color codes that show at a glance the overall health value of the product. However, reading and understanding nutrition labels is the most powerful thing you can do to compare what you know your own needs are against the general recommendations. Understanding label language and laws is very helpful in being able to determine what's best for you.

Food terms deciphered

THESE WORDS MAY APPEAR TO BE DESCRIBING UNHEALTHY ADDITIVES, BUT THEY ARE ALTERNATIVE NAMES FOR HEALTHY ADDITIONS THAT WILL DO YOU NO HARM.

Tocopherols: Vitamin E, used as a preservative to prevent the oils and fats in a product from going rancid

Locust bean: From the carob tree, used to thicken items such as yogurt and cream cheese

Pyridoxine hydrochloride: Vitamin B6

Calcium pantothenate: Calcium and vitamin B5

Inulin: Extracted from chicory root, inulin is a source of fiber that can also be substituted for fat in foods

Ferrous gluconate: A source of Iron

1,25 dihydroxycholicalciferol: Vitamin D

Ascorbic acid: Vitamin C

Ascorbyl palmitate: Vitamin C attached to fat

Acetic acid: Vinegar, a food preservative

SHOULD I CHOOSE ORGANIC?

It has long been debated whether organic food is better than that produced conventionally. Demand for organic is increasing, but it remains a question of personal taste and priorities.

THE EVIDENCE

Organic food is produced without using synthetic fertilizers and pesticides. Google "organic food," and you will be bombarded with a mix of foods and products marketed as must-have foods for your health. The truth behind the claims is very different. The reality is that there is still limited research and next to no large-scale high-quality studies looking into organic food, although we do have a handful of small-scale studies with very mixed results. One review of 233 studies concluded that there isn't enough evidence to suggest that we all consume organic food for nutritional benefits. Apart from the use of pesticides, crop quality is also dependent on other factors such as the weather, soil quality, when crops are harvested, and, for animal products, the product is affected by the overall diet and lifestyle of the animal. Even the handling of produce by humans can impact the finished product.

THE ENVIRONMENT

What is generally accepted is that the production of organic food is beneficial for the environment. Organic farming reduces the use of synthetic pesticides (although some natural pesticides may still be allowed). Farming this way on a large scale would potentially increase the quality of our food, build better soil health, increase biodiversity and biomass, and be better for environmental protection.

PESTICIDES

While organic produce is grown without the use of pesticides, nonorganic foods may contain some residue of pesticides, although they are often within safe limits for consumption. Every year, the Environmental Working Group (EWG) releases a list of the 12 nonorganic fruits and vegetables highest in pesticide residues. It is important to note that this list is not backed by trusted food bodies across the world, and there is an argument that the list is creating fear for the public when consuming healthy food items. While it is true pesticides can build up if consumed in excess over time, the benefits of consuming the food outweighs this, and most pesticides can be removed by simply washing your fruits and vegetables.

Some types of food that cannot be washed, such as oats, may still contain pesticides so may be worth buying organic. Levels of the harmful pesticide glyphosate that was prevalent in oat-based products is on the decline, according to recent tests.

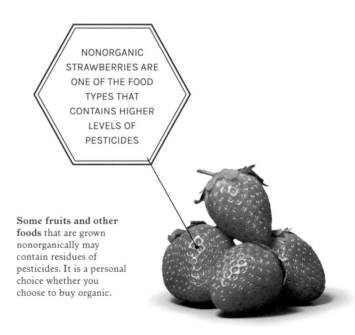

NONORGANIC STRAWBERRIES ARE ONE OF THE FOOD TYPES THAT CONTAINS HIGHER LEVELS OF PESTICIDES

Some fruits and other foods that are grown nonorganically may contain residues of pesticides. It is a personal choice whether you choose to buy organic.

LEVELS OF PESTICIDES

LOWER LEVELS

AVOCADOS	KIWI FRUIT
CORN	CABBAGE
PINEAPPLE	MUSHROOMS
ONIONS	MANGOES
PAPAYA	SWEET POTATOES
PEAS (FROZEN)	WATERMELON
ASPARAGUS	CARROTS

HIGHER LEVELS

STRAWBERRIES	APPLES
SPINACH	GRAPES
KALE	BELL PEPPERS
CABBAGE	CHILLI PEPPERS
PEACHES	CHERRIES
PEARS	BLUEBERRIES
NECTARINES	GREEN BEANS

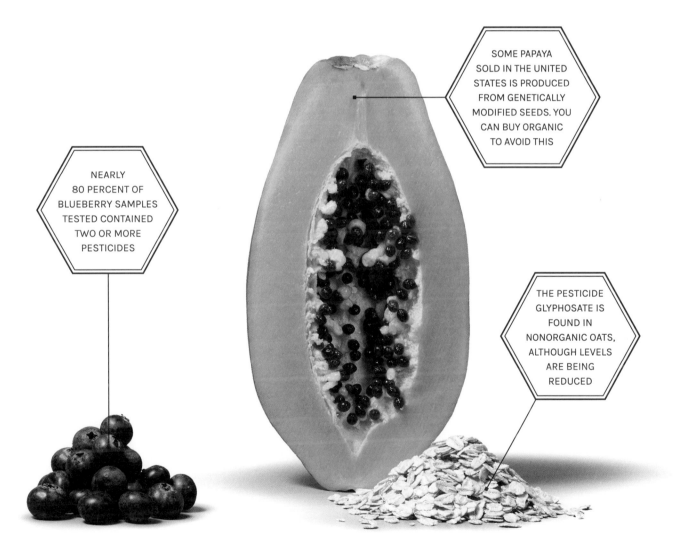

SOME PAPAYA SOLD IN THE UNITED STATES IS PRODUCED FROM GENETICALLY MODIFIED SEEDS. YOU CAN BUY ORGANIC TO AVOID THIS

NEARLY 80 PERCENT OF BLUEBERRY SAMPLES TESTED CONTAINED TWO OR MORE PESTICIDES

THE PESTICIDE GLYPHOSATE IS FOUND IN NONORGANIC OATS, ALTHOUGH LEVELS ARE BEING REDUCED

HOW DO I ACHIEVE CREAMINESS IN A DISH?

If opting to reduce or eliminate dairy from your diet, the texture and appearance of some foods may be different from what you're used to, but there are many ways to still achieve the rich, creamy mouthfeel that dairy ingredients provide.

Many cultures around the world traditionally consume little milk and cheese and cook delicious food and beverages without the need to add dairy at all. Here are a few suggestions of foods that you can use in vegan or dairy-free cooking that will create a creamy taste and texture.

● **Coconut** is a common addition to curries and sauces in the kitchen. Coconut milk can be used in curries to create a creamy texture. It is fatty in a similar way to cow's milk and can also be used in soups and desserts. Coconut cream has a thicker consistency and can be chilled and whipped into a stiff and creamy whipped form. It solidifies when chilled and so is useful for icings and ice-cream alternatives. It is worth remembering that coconut milk, coconut cream, and coconut oil contain relatively high levels of saturated fat, which should be consumed in moderation. Some research has suggested that the saturated fat (MCTs) in coconuts may be metabolized differently from other saturated fats, although more work is needed in this area before these claims can be proved. Eating these

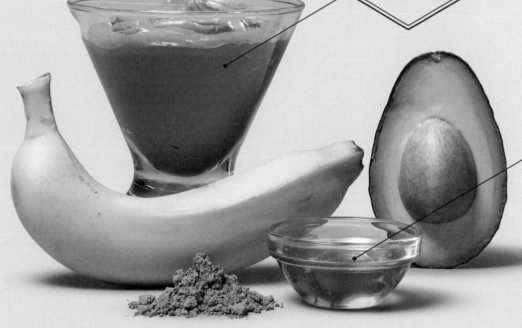

MOUSSE CAN BE MADE BY BLENDING AVOCADOS, ALMOND MILK, AGAVE NECTAR, AND CACAO POWDER

ADD MAPLE SYRUP TO OLIVE OIL TO CREATE A CREAMY DRESSING

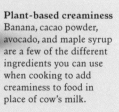

Plant-based creaminess
Banana, cacao powder, avocado, and maple syrup are a few of the different ingredients you can use when cooking to add creaminess to food in place of cow's milk.

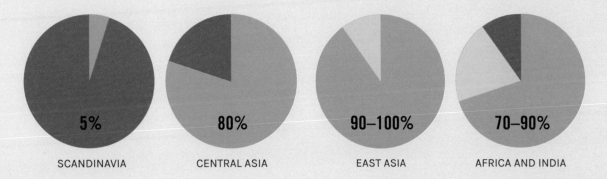

LACTOSE INTOLERANT

Percentages of populations around the
world who are unable to eat dairy foods.
Many cultures have found ways to prepare
and cook foods without using cow's milk.

ingredients as part of a balanced, healthy diet is
recommended (see box below, right).

● **Tahini** is a creamy, smooth paste made from
sesame seeds. It contains a high proportion of
healthy unsaturated fats and can be used as a spread
and/or drizzled over salads and stirred into soups.
Tahini can also be added to smoothies to increase
their creaminess, and it is a key ingredient in
hummus, imparting a creamy texture.

● **Avocado** can be blended to a creamy consistency
and used as a cold pasta sauce and is a source of
healthy monounsaturated fats, including oleic acid,
which can help with heart health. Avocado can also
be used in place of butter or mayonnaise and in some
cold desserts, such as cacao mousse (shown left).

● **Nuts and nut butters** are a popular addition to
food for their health benefits (see pp.128–129), but
peanut butter especially is used widely in savory and
sweet dishes for its creaminess. Try using peanut
butter in your soups as a thickener and in chilies and
stews. Peanut butter can also be added to dressings
to enhance their creaminess, and often tastes good
with Thai flavors like lime and chili sauce. It can also
be used to make a rich icing on a cake. Try it paired
with dark chocolate cake or biscuits. Cashews can be
soaked and blended to provide a creamy sauce and
are a source of various nutrients, including

magnesium, iron, manganese, copper, and zinc. Vegan
cheese sauces are often made using cashews.

Other ingredients you can try include potatoes,
which make a creamy mash or soup base. Frozen
bananas (shown opposite) can be used to make
creamy ice cream, and you can also blend and whip
silken tofu or puréed white beans to create creamy
white sauces. Vegan creams and spread alternatives,
often with a soy, nut, or coconut base, can also be
bought to add to your recipes.

What are MCTs?

**MEDIUM-CHAIN TRIGYLDERIDES (MCTs) ARE A
TYPE OF SATURATED FAT.**

Coconut oil is high in saturated fat composed of
MCTs. Some studies have suggested that MCTs may
have a positive impact on weight management by
increasing feelings of fullness and may enhance fat
oxidation (energy release from fat). Triglycerides
with short- or medium-chain fatty acids have a
higher proportion of carbon and hydrogen in the
molecule and so have fewer calories than
triglycerides with longer chain lengths. More
research is needed before any claims can be made,
and as a general rule, we need to keep our intake of
saturated fat to a minimum.

HOW CAN I RECREATE "MEATY" FLAVORS IN A DISH?

Meat has a distinct flavor, but scientists and chefs have been exploring ways to recreate the taste and textures of meat in dishes without using the key ingredient itself.

The savory taste of meat comes from its umami flavor—a blend of sugar, fat, and protein that is highly appealing to the palate. Usually, meat is aged for a few hours, during which time proteins break down and release amino acids. Of these amino acids and other molecules that are released, glutamate, inosinate, and guanylate give meat its umami savoriness. Cooking the meat causes the molecules in meat to break down further, and the heat chemically alters many of these molecules.

UMAMI

To get meaty flavors in plant-based dishes, you can add umami-rich ingredients such as mushrooms, soy sauce, miso, nutritional yeast, tomatoes, and seaweed. Umami is one of the five basic flavors alongside sweet, salty, bitter, and sour. The umami taste comes from the prescence of glutamic acid, a naturally occurring amino acid found in protein-rich foods like meat, cheese, and stocks. Parmesan cheese contains 1,680mg of glutamic acid per 100g, and soy

Rich flavors Try adding ingredients such as mushrooms, seaweed, or tomatoes for a depth and richness of flavor.

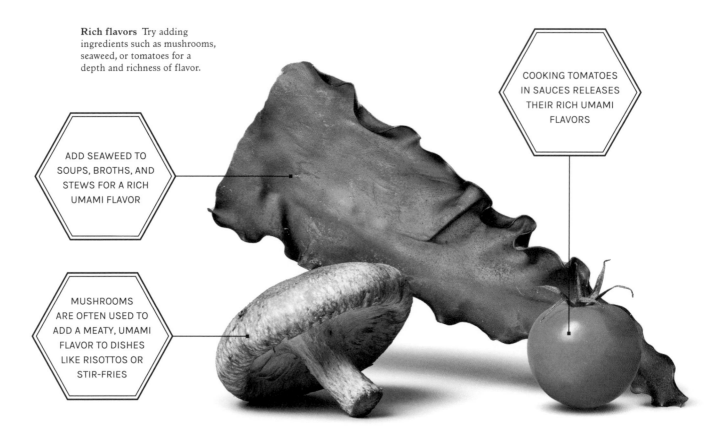

ADD SEAWEED TO SOUPS, BROTHS, AND STEWS FOR A RICH UMAMI FLAVOR

COOKING TOMATOES IN SAUCES RELEASES THEIR RICH UMAMI FLAVORS

MUSHROOMS ARE OFTEN USED TO ADD A MEATY, UMAMI FLAVOR TO DISHES LIKE RISOTTOS OR STIR-FRIES

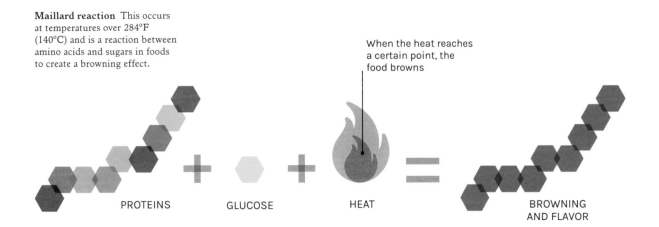

Maillard reaction This occurs at temperatures over 284°F (140°C) and is a reaction between amino acids and sugars in foods to create a browning effect.

When the heat reaches a certain point, the food browns

PROTEINS + GLUCOSE + HEAT = BROWNING AND FLAVOR

sauce has 782mg per 100g. Monosodium glutamate (MSG) is an artificial flavoring made from sodium and glutamate that is often used to add a meaty, umami taste to processed foods. While MSG cannot be eaten in large amounts by some people, it has been shown to be safe for human consumption.

CARAMELIZATION AND THE MAILLARD REACTION

Enzymatic browning is when enzymes chemically alter the food (this is also what happens when fruits ripen). There are two types of nonenzymatic browning: the Maillard reaction and caramelization. A Maillard reaction is a chemical reaction between proteins and sugars that are transformed by heat to create distinct flavors, aromas, and a brown color that makes food enticing. The reaction happens between reducing sugars and amino acids at temperatures of 230°F (110°C) to 329°F (165°C) and creates complex compounds that culminate in a distinct flavor, aroma, and taste. A Maillard reaction is also affected by pH and temperature.

Caramelization is a reaction that happens at higher temperatures than the Maillard reaction of 320°F (160°C) and above. It involves the breakdown of sugars to create the sweetness, distinct brown color, flavor, and aroma of these foods. The brown char on grilled meat is due to caramelization, and it gives the meat a slightly nutty flavor.

ADDING "MEAT" FLAVORS

There are a number of ways you can try to recreate some of the flavors caused by caramelization and the Maillard reaction. For a grilled meat taste, some restaurants now use liquid smoke, smoked salt, and kelp. Additional flavors such as smoked paprika, barbecue sauce, mustard, curry powder, and teriyaki sauce also work well. You can also now buy vegan gravy granules, which mimic the taste of meat, to add to your recipes. Scientists have been exploring meat alternatives for years, and the ingredients of new burgers and other meat items now taste virtually identical to meat (see pp.46–47). It is estimated that the consumption of these alternatives may save 250,000 animal lives each year.

ADDING "MEATY" TEXTURE

Considering the texture of food can also help replicate a meaty taste. For a beeflike texture, you could try using either seitan (see pp.120–121) or tofu (see pp.118–119), and for a chicken texture, try a mushroom/jackfruit combination. Vegetables such as eggplant and lentils can be added to many recipes in place of meat to provide taste and a "meaty" texture. Seasoning vegetables also adds a taste to accompany the texture. To do this, you can add vegetable stock and vegan Worcestershire sauce (check the labels to determine whether they are vegan), or you can use tomato purée or ketchup.

WHAT TECHNIQUES ARE NEEDED FOR PLANT-BASED BAKING?

The science of food is both intricate and fascinating—that perfect combination of fat and sugar to satisfy our taste buds or the texture of that muffin or cake. It is entirely possible to bake without the use of animal produce and still get the same taste and textures.

For thousands of years, eggs and butter have been used in baking. Eggs act as binding agents due to the presence of specific proteins in the egg whites, which coagulate during baking. Proteins in eggs also contribute to the leavening process of some baked goods, whereby air is trapped and expands during baking, providing a lift or rise to the goods. Eggs also add moisture to batters and doughs, and their yolks contains emulsifiers that blend fats and liquids. Butter adds flavor, richness, and creaminess to baked goods, and its fat helps create a crumbly and flaky texture in baking.

REPLACING EGGS

Traditionally, eggs are used in baking to help bind ingredients, to thicken, emulsify, build volume, stabilize, and provide unique colors and flavors. Although eggs are nutritious and versatile (see pp.54–55), you can replace them with plant ingredients in your favorite baked goods (see below). Cornstarch can also act as an egg replacement to provide the binding and moisture-retaining properties they typically provide. Mix together 1 tablespoon of cornstarch with 3 tablespoons of water to replace one egg.

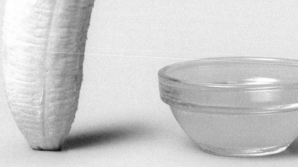

Egg substitutions

Eggs provide a wide range of attributes beneficial for baking. Unfortunately, due to the complexity of their nutritional composition, there is no perfect substitute for eggs that can mimic their binding, volumizing, emulsifying, leavening, and thickening properties.

½
BANANA

= ONE EGG

Peel and mash the banana to a smooth consistency. Half a banana usually equates to one egg.

3 tbsp
AQUAFABA

= ONE EGG

For aquafaba (see pp.126–127), whisk the juice from a can of chickpeas. 1 tbsp is needed for an egg yolk, 2 tbsp are needed for an egg white, and 3 tbsp for one egg.

This works particularly well in cookie and cake recipes. It can also be used as a thickening agent in sauces, puddings, and dessert-like recipes where it provides a smooth and velvety texture. Another great alternative is aquafaba, which is made from the juice from a can of chickpeas (see pp.126–127). However, none of these ingredients work particularly well as an emulsifier.

BUTTER SUBSTITUTIONS

When replacing butter with a vegan alternative, you may need to add vegetable fat or shortening (solid fat made from vegetable oils such as soybean) in order to achieve the correct texture. You can use three-quarters vegan butter and one-quarter vegetable shortening or experiment with different plant butters to see how they work in your recipe.

When replacing butter in a recipe with a vegan alternative, the choice of substitute is crucial as dairy-free alternatives have different structures.

Traditional dairy butter contains a unique combination of fat, water, and milk solids that contributes to the flavor, texture, and the way it functions within different recipes. Plant-based alternatives to butter do not have the same composition as dairy butter, which may have implications for flavor, texture, and functionality. The use of vegan butter for making buttercream icing can work, but it may take some experimenting to find out which one works best.

WHAT ABOUT MARGARINE?

Many think margarine and vegan butter are the same thing, and when looking at ingredient lists, it may appear that way. However, margarine may contain milk solids in the form of buttermilk, whereas vegan butter is 100 percent plant-based. If the margarine in question is labeled as being vegan and plant-based, then it usually contains vegetable oils made from soybeans, rapeseed, or sunflower seeds.

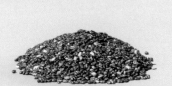

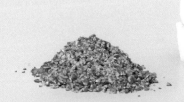

1 tbsp
CHIA SEEDS +

3 tbsp WATER = ONE EGG

For chia seeds, mix 1 tbsp of chia seeds and 3 tbsp of water and set aside until gloopy. This gives a similar consistency to one egg.

1 tbsp
GROUND FLAXSEED +

3 tbsp WATER = ONE EGG

For a flaxseed egg, mix 1 tbsp of ground flaxseed with 3 tbsp of water and let soak until gloopy.

8oz
SILKEN TOFU

= ONE EGG

Silken tofu can also work in dense, moist, or savory recipes; 8oz (225g) of silken tofu can create the effect of one egg.

HOW DO I COOK FOR MAXIMUM NUTRITION?

It is important to consider the way you prepare and cook plant foods. There are a variety of different cooking methods available to us, and each has a different impact on the nutritional value of the food we then eat.

Aside from choosing ingredients that meet our health needs, cooking methods can impact how many nutrients they provide.

TIPS FOR COOKING AND CHOOSING FOOD

Here are some tips for cooking at home:

● Avoid unhealthy cooking methods such as deep-frying and cooking for long periods at high temperatures and opt for stir-fries, microwaved, or steamed vegetables. Don't overcook your food and eat vegetables with a crunch as they will retain more nutrition this way.

● Choose fresh or frozen vegetables because canned and pickled vegetables can sometimes be packaged with salt (check the ingredients list). Fruits and vegetables are picked at peak ripeness and often frozen within hours, locking in nutrients and flavor. Generally, frozen foods retain their vitamins and minerals, and there is no difference in the carbohydrate, protein, and fat content compared with fresh produce. In some cases, frozen foods actually contain more vitamins and minerals because fresh foods lose nutrients if stored, while freezing preserves them.

COOKING OILS

All oils have different characteristics and therefore meet different needs. It is important to match the oil's heat tolerance with the temperature used. The "smoke point" of cooking oils is the point when oils

Cooking methods

Some of the more common ways of cooking with their advantages and disadvantages.

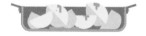

ROASTING

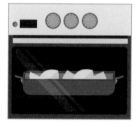

OVEN COOKED

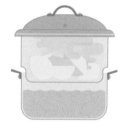

STEAMING

PROS: Many foods can be roasted, including vegetables, pulses, and meats.

CONS: Protein content of certain seeds may decrease as roasting temperature increases.

PROS: Can cook larger amounts of food at the same time. If cooking for shorter periods of time, fewer nutrients are lost.

CONS: Tender vegetables may lose micronutrients.

PROS: Gentle steaming retains nutrients, texture, and color and doesn't add calories as you don't need to use oil.

CONS: It is easy to overcook vegetables, leading to nutrient loss.

start to burn or smoke (see p.155). If you heat oil past this point, it will affect the flavor, nutrients will degrade, and harmful compounds called free radicals may be released.

VITAMIN CONTENT

Water-soluble vitamins are easily destroyed during preparation and cooking. This happens when they are exposed to heat or water, so boiling vegetables can result in vitamins dissolving in the water. Scrub vegetables instead of peeling them, as many nutrients found close to the skin can be lost. Better still, leave vegetable skins on during cooking to retain their nutrients. Microwave or steam instead of boiling to cut down on vitamin and mineral loss. You can also eat many vegetables raw for maximum vitamin intake. Fat-soluble vitamins are more stable, although they can still be affected by overcooking. Some nutrients work with oils to improve availability. For example, cooking spinach in a little oil can help make fat-soluble vitamin A more available once absorbed by the body. You can also prepare some foods without cooking traditionally. Light pickling with an acid (vinegar) can make raw chopped vegetables more palatable.

Cooking oils

WHEN CHOOSING AN OIL, YOU NEED TO CONSIDER THE DISH YOU'RE PREPARING AND HOW YOU'RE COOKING IT.

EXTRA-VIRGIN OLIVE OIL
Use for salad dressings, marinades, dipping sauces, and light sautéing.

AVOCADO OIL
Good for cooking at high temperatures, deep-frying, pan-frying, sautéing, and stir-frying

RAPESEED/CANOLA OIL
Ideal for deep-frying, pan-frying, searing, roasting, and high temperature cooking.

PEANUT OIL (UNREFINED)
Good for sauces or dressings.

PEANUT OIL (REFINED)
Can be used at high temperatures for deep frying and pan-frying

SUNFLOWER OIL
Neutral flavor, can be used for frying.

SOYBEAN OIL
Soybean oil is a good source of omega-6 fatty acids. Use for frying, sautéing, baking, salad dressings, and marinades.

FLAXSEED OIL
Add to smoothies, salad dressings, or drizzle over finished dishes to enhance flavor.

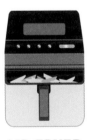

AIR FRYER

PROS: Less oil used, lower fat intakes, and can lower acrylamide production by up to 90% (see pp.154–155).

CONS: As much less oil is needed, fewer healthy fats may be consumed, which may affect fat-soluble vitamin absorption. The benefits of consuming extra-virgin olive oil may be lost.

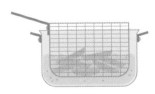

FRYING

PROS: More oil is used, which improves the color, flavor, and crispiness of foods.

CONS: Relatively high oil content and high temperatures can increase the risk of acrylamide formation (a carcinogenous product). Water-soluble vitamins degraded.

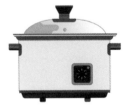

SLOW COOKER

PROS: Gentle cooking at low temperatures means food keeps its nutrients. Some water-soluble vitamins are retained.

CONS: Not suitable for foods such as delicate vegetables. If left too long, food can be overcooked.

154

SHOULD I BE USING
AN AIR FRYER?

Air fryers are very popular and promise to cut cooking times and use less energy than conventional ovens. They produce less waste and use less energy than other frying techniques, but are they healthier than other ways of cooking?

While you certainly do not need an air fryer to cook meals, there are benefits in terms of speed of cooking and the amount of oil needed to cook the food.

LESS OIL AND FAT

When using an air fryer to cook, you don't need to use as much oil as you would if you were frying in a pan or deep frying the same meal. Instead of placing food into oil, the air fryer circulates hot air around the food, which gives it a crispy texture. Less oil is healthier than frying as it results in less fat, as well as potentially a crispier texture, so it is a quick and healthier way to fry, and you can cut the calories by 80 percent. This is not always beneficial when it comes to the absorption of fat-soluble vitamins, but

Lower acrylamide

ACRYLAMIDE IS A CHEMICAL COMPOUND THAT MAY INCREASE YOUR RISK OF CANCER.
Compared to cooking in oil, air frying helps lower levels of acrylamide, which is found in starchy foods, like potatoes. Acrylamide is a chemical compound that can form naturally in starchy foods during high-temperature cooking processes such as frying, roasting, or baking. It is produced when sugars and amino acids react in the presence of heat. This compound has raised concerns regarding the potential increased risk of cancer, and so reducing its levels is understood to be beneficial to general health.

it may be helpful for those trying to look after their health by reducing fat intake.

HOW DO AIR FRYERS WORK?

Air fryers cook food via convection, with use of a high-powered fan and a heating element. The fan circulates hot air rapidly throughout the cooking chamber, which contains the food, creating a convection current. In air fryers, air molecules near the heating element gain energy as they become heated. These molecules become less dense, rise, and create an upward flow. As these energized molecules move away from the heat source, they gradually release their energy, cool down, and become denser again, causing a downward flow. This process is the underlying cause of convection currents, which facilitates the transfer of heat from the hot air to the food.

This circulating hot (energized) air cooks the food from all angles and ensures even heat distribution, reducing the chance of one side of the food catching or burning. A constant hot air flow allows the food to become crispy and browned, similar to traditional frying methods, yet requires significantly less oil. Air frying is, therefore, highly advantageous as it not only enhances the texture of food, but it also substantially reduces the cooking times compared to traditional frying methods.

MORE NUTRITION

We know that if food is exposed to heat for shorter amounts of time when cooking, it will lose fewer nutrients, such as vitamins and phytochemicals (see pp.152–153). With a shorter cooking time, air fried foods are likely to retain more nutrients than when using alternative cooking methods. However, air fryers can come with a high price tag, and while it is a good alternative to conventional frying methods, there is no evidence to suggest that this way of cooking is healthier than boiling or steaming.

WHICH OIL SHOULD I USE?

Different cooking oils are used for different methods of cooking depending on their flavor, which may depend on your personal choice and their smoke point. This is the temperature at which the oil begins to break down, creating smoke, which can affect the taste of the food and release harmful compounds.

Monounsaturated oils such as olive oil, avocado oil, and peanut oil are a good choice from a health point of view because they contain healthy fats. **Olive oil** can be used in an air fryer because it remains stable at high temperatures, with a fairly high smoke point. There are many types of olive oils available on the market, labeled as "light olive oil," "pure olive oil," "extra light olive oil," and just "olive oil," which have high smoke points but are heavily refined, meaning they lose the nutritional compounds that extra-virgin olive oil has. If you are cooking at less than 392°F (200°C) in the oven or air fryer, then extra-virgin olive oil is the best option as it contains the healthy polyphenol compounds lost through processing.

For temperatures over 392°F (200°C), **avocado oil** is a good option because it has a higher smoke point than extra-virgin olive oil. **Refined peanut oil** has a high smoke point of about 450°F (232°C), making it good for air frying, deep-frying, pan-frying, and sautéing. **Canola oil** (also known as rapeseed oil) is another good choice for air frying because it is high in monounsaturated fats (omega-9) and polyunsaturated fatty acids (omega-3 and -6) and is also an excellent source of vitamin E.

Polyunsaturated oils, including **sunflower oil** and **soybean oil**, have high smoke points, which means they are suited to high-heat cooking. Most vegetable and seed oils are high in omega-6, which just needs to be balanced with omega-3 (see pp.102–103).

HIGH HEAT THESE OILS CAN BE USED FOR FRYING, STIR-FRYING, AND GRILLING	520°F (270°C) Avocado oil (refined) 465°F (240°C) Light olive oil (refined) 450°F (232°C) Peanut oil (refined) 440°F (226°C) Sunflower oil 430°F (221°C) Almond oil 428°F (220°C) Vegetable oil (refined)
MEDIUM HEAT USE THESE OILS FOR BAKING AND FRYING	425°F (218°C) Hazelnut oil 420°F (215°C) Grapeseed oil 410°F (210°C) Sesame oil (refined) 400°F (204°C) Canola oil (refined) 400°F (204°C) Vegetable oil 375°F (190°C) Extra-virgin olive oil
LOW HEAT TRY THESE OILS FOR GENTLE FRYING	350°F (177°C) Coconut oil (unrefined) 350°F (177°C) Sesame oil (unrefined) 320°F (160°C) Sunflower oil (unrefined) 320°F (160°C) Peanut oil (unrefined) 320°F (160°C) Walnut oil (unrefined) 300°F (149°C) Hempseed oil
NO HEAT USE FOR SALAD DRESSINGS	225°F (107°C) Almond oil 225°F (107°C) Flaxseed oil

OIL SMOKE POINTS

Different oils start to burn at a range of temperatures, so you need to choose one that works for your cooking method.

Saturated oils remain moderately stable during cooking, although they are high in saturated fat. **Refined coconut oil** is good for high-heat cooking, including air frying and stir-frying. **Unrefined coconut oil** has a lower smoke point and is best for baking and low-medium heat cooking, such as sautéing. **Palm oil** can be used to cook at high temperatures such as deep-frying but should be limited in consumption due to its high saturated fat content. It has also caused a negative impact on the environment through deforestation.

SHOULD I BE USING A PRESSURE COOKER?

Pressure cooking is the process of cooking food using steam at a very high pressure and water or a water-based cooling liquid. The pressure limits boiling, resulting in cooking temperatures that are higher and food that cooks more quickly.

HOW IT WORKS

Cooking generally involves raising the temperature of food until chemical reactions take place, like those that break down the tough tissue in meat or soften the starch in vegetables. Those reactions usually happen faster at higher temperatures.

A pressure cooker works by trapping the steam formed by cooking food in water inside a steel chamber. The higher cooking temperature inside a sealed pressure cooker means that the food cooks faster without burning. The accelerated cooking process in a pressure cooker can be attributed to

boiling point elevation, which is driven by the increased atmospheric pressure inside the sealed cooker. Under normal conditions, water boils at 212°F (100°C); however, the increased pressure within a pressure cooker increases its boiling point, which allows the water to reach higher temperatures before turning to steam. This causes a faster transfer of heat to the food, resulting in increased molecular activity in the food. Ultimately, the heightened temperature and pressure inside this type of cooker contributes to the breakdown of complex nutrients such as starch and protein at a significantly faster rate than other cooking methods.

The same phenomenon explains why cooking at high altitudes is different to cooking at sea level. Air pressure decreases as you move higher above sea

Cooking under pressure

As temperatures in a sealed pressure cooker are high you can cook faster without burning food. Limited evaporation also means you don't lose flavor.

PRESSURE COOKER IS HEATED

Food is placed in the sealed container and liquid is added, then the cooker is plugged in or placed on a burner.

STEAM BUILDS UP

As the liquid inside the pressure cooker heats, steam collects in the sealed vessel of the cooker.

TEMPERATURE RISES

Energized steam molecules cannot escape, causing pressure to increase and, as a result, the boiling temperature.

level. At lower pressures, water boils at a lower temperature and so food will take longer to cook. Under these conditions, a pressure cooker can raise the pressure and the boiling point and cook food faster. At the same time, the moisture is retained because the water cannot evaporate.

The sealed environment of the pressure cooker means that the cooker retains moisture and limits accessibility to oxygen. This means that the combustion reactions necessary for burning are inhibited, preventing burning.

GOOD FOR PLANT-BASED DIETS

There is mixed evidence as to whether pressure cooking has superior results to other cooking methods in terms of nutrient retention. However, it is a fast method of cooking, so you may choose to use it for time-saving purposes. For plant-based eating, this way of cooking can be extremely useful because pressure cookers simplify the preparation process for cooking beans and pulses, removing the need for presoaking. This time-efficient method makes following a legume-rich diet accessible and appealing. Cooking plant-based dishes such as risottos can be done in half the time in a pressure

cooker. Pressure cookers can also save money on fuel costs as they cook more quickly than other methods.

ANTINUTRIENTS AND PRESSURE COOKING

Pressure cooking has been found to increase starch digestibility and improve reduction in antinutrients when cooking beans. Antinutrients are naturally occurring compounds commonly found in plants, which can interfere with the absorption or utilization of nutrients in the body. One example of this is phytic acid, which is found in legumes, which negatively impacts the absorption of iron in the small intestine. Although the term "antinutrient" may sound negative, it is important to understand that they are not all inherently "bad." In fact, tannins, antinutrients found in tea and coffee, are known for their antioxidant properties.

ARE THERE ANY CONS?

Pressure cookers are less effective than steaming or lightly boiling more delicate vegetables as they use such a high heat that it quickly destroys their nutrients. To avoid this, you can adjust the timing of the additions of food into the cooker, adding more delicate ingredients later in the cooking process. With pressure cooker recipes, all cooking times should be taken only from when the level of pressure is reached, at which point you should lower the heat but try to maintain the same level of pressure for the time stated. This can involve turning the heat up and down during the cooking process or moving the pan to a different size stove burner.

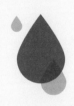

LACK OF
EVAPORATION

The food cooks quickly, retaining nutrients, and doesn't lose flavor through evaporation.

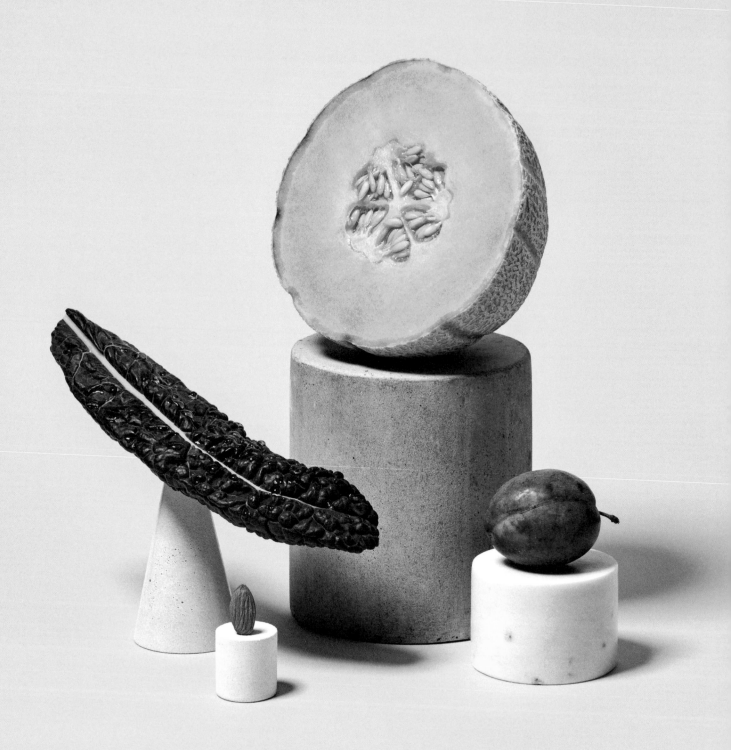

PLANT-BASED NUTRITION FOR LIFE AND HEALTH

IS A PLANT-BASED DIET SAFE DURING PREGNANCY?

Pregnancy is often a time when diet becomes a focus for women who want to nourish their baby and themselves. The type of dietary choices a woman makes will directly impact her nutrition status and that of the fetus.

If you are pregnant or are considering becoming pregnant, your nutrition is an important factor to consider, whether you're eating a plant-based diet or not. A mother's diet is what sustains and helps the development of her unborn baby, and so it is important to get the right nutrition before, during, and after birth. Recommendations for diet during pregnancy vary around the world, but most countries consider a plant-based diet to be a safe way of eating throughout pregnancy and lactation.

NUTRITIONAL DEFICIENCIES

While plant-based diets carry many benefits, if they are not carefully planned and well balanced, then there may be a risk of nutritional deficiencies both for mother and fetus. It is likely that in addition to the folic acid and vitamin D recommended to all pregnant women, further supplementation will be required. If you are plant-based or vegan, you also need to make sure you are getting enough iron, vitamin B12, calcium, omega-3, and iodine, as these are the nutrients that are often found more easily in a diet that includes meat and dairy foods.

If you think you may not be meeting the daily requirements of these nutrients, it's best to seek advice from a qualified healthcare professional as you may need to supplement your diet, depending on your individual needs (see pp.96–113).

THE RESEARCH

There is little research in the area of nutrition and plant-based eating during pregnancy. However, there is some evidence for a reduction in gestational hypertension, including preeclampsia when

Eating right

If you are pregnant, make sure that you are getting enough of these food types, which have been linked to healthy brain growth for growing fetuses.

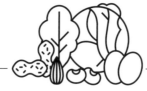

CHOLINE

FOOD SOURCES

EGGS | CRUCIFEROUS VEGETABLES (BRASSICAS) | NUTS | LEGUMES

SHOULD I SUPPLEMENT?

Supplementing with twice the recommended amount of choline (450mg/day) in the third trimester of pregnancy may improve speed of processing in infants; especially important for plant-based eaters.

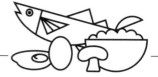

VITAMIN D

FOOD SOURCES

FATTY FISH | EGG YOLKS | FORTIFIED FOODS | MUSHROOMS GROWN IN SUNLIGHT

SHOULD I SUPPLEMENT?

If you get little or no sun exposure, take a daily 400 IU supplement all year. Deficiency in pregnancy has been linked to an increased risk of a child developing ADHD and a reduction in cognition and language abilities (see pp.104–105).

Development of the brain This is
heavily reliant on the diet of the mother
in the first few weeks of pregnancy.

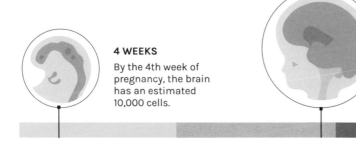

4 WEEKS
By the 4th week of
pregnancy, the brain
has an estimated
10,000 cells.

24 WEEKS
By the 24th week,
the child's brain
contains 10
billion cells.

KEY

1st trimester
(0–13 weeks)

2nd trimester
(14–26 weeks)

3rd trimester
(27–40 weeks)

following a diet rich in plant-based foods, such as
fruits, vegetables, whole grains, vegetable oils, nuts,
and legumes. Those who eat plant-based diets are
also associated with a reduced risk of other
pregnancy-related issues such as preterm birth,
gestational diabetes mellitus, and excessive
gestational weight gain. There is also some limited
evidence that suggests a plant-based diet is linked
with a reduced risk of postpartum depression. This
may be due to the potential benefits of plant-based
diets related to obesity and gestational diabetes,
although more research is needed to confirm a link.
Plant-based diets during pregnancy may reduce the
onset of diseases that affect the baby, such as

pediatric wheezing, diabetes, neural tube defects,
face and mouth clefts, and some pediatric tumors.

IN SUMMARY

Plant-based diets are safe during pregnancy,
but they may require careful planning and
supplementation, with a key focus on specific
nutrients such as vitamin B12, calcium, iron, and
vitamin D, to help avoid certain deficiencies and
support the optimal growth and development of
a baby. We need more research and a standard
definition of a plant-based diet itself, as dietary
habits vary from individual to individual and
do not consider lifestyle factors.

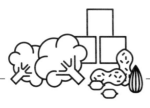

IRON

FOOD SOURCES

BROCCOLI | TOFU | NUTS | BEANS | DRIED FRUIT

SHOULD I SUPPLEMENT?

Up to 50 percent of pregnant women are iron
deficient, which can cause neural issues in the
fetus; those with gestational diabetes are more
at risk. Iron in the third trimester is
especially important (see pp.98–99).

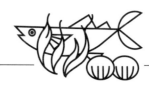

OMEGA-3 DHA

FOOD SOURCES

FISH AND SEAFOOD | SEAWEED AND ALGAE

SHOULD I SUPPLEMENT?

A fetus's needs increase sharply in the third trimester
since the brain consists of fatty acids. Studies
suggest DHA supplements could give babies better
memory, attention, and verbal skills and a lower risk
of neurological disorders (see pp.102–103).

IS PLANT-BASED WEANING SAFE FOR BABIES?

Traditionally there are many ways to wean a baby, but over the past decade or so a vegetable-led approach has become popular. Some statistics even suggest that adopting a vegetable-first approach may increase the likelihood of your child accepting them as they grow older.

There are different approaches to introducing food: baby-led, spoon-fed, or a combination of both. Baby-led weaning involves giving your baby finger foods and letting them feed themselves, while spoon-feeding involves feeding them puréed or mashed foods such as veggie purées, rice, and fruit. There is no right or wrong way; it is a personal choice and will be viewed differently in different cultures. However, research shows a combination approach helps promote autonomous feeding, oral development, and appetite control. If you start with purées, offer finger foods alongside to promote the practice of self-feeding by at least nine months of age.

EARLY EXPOSURE TO VEGETABLES

The benefits to plant-based weaning are emerging, and it is now common to start with vegetables over baby rice or other baby foods. The theories behind this make a lot of sense—starting with bitter-tasting vegetables as opposed to the more acceptable sweeter foods for babies may result in a child who readily accepts a variety of vegetables. Studies have shown that early exposure to vegetables may increase the likelihood of a child accepting vegetables as they age. Some research suggests that between six to 12 months is when babies are most likely to try and accept new foods, a time often referred to as a "window of opportunity," which makes it a good time to offer a wide variety of foods. Fiber found in vegetables can also help with more regular bowel movements and prevent constipation.

IRON

Babies accumulate iron in the womb and store enough to last for the first four to six months of life, after which it is important they begin to get iron from their diet. Breast milk is low in iron (around 0.3g/l), and formula also contains a low amount, which is why diet is important. Babies need 11mg of iron a day between the ages of 7 to 12 months. Foods rich in vitamin C, such as citrus fruits, strawberries, raspberries, cauliflower, and potatoes promote iron absorption. Studies have shown that vitamin C can counteract inhibitors found in plants like phytic acid (which make plant iron less bioavailable) and increase iron absorption by 3–6 times. It is complex to try and figure out exactly how much iron your baby is getting each day, and public health guidelines suggest that it is not possible for infants to attain all of their iron requirements from whole foods alone (especially if breastfed). Adding fortified foods, such

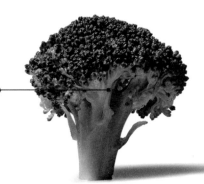

BROCCOLI
SOME RESEARCH SUGGESTS WEANING WITH BITTER FLAVORS MAKES THEM MORE ACCEPTED LATER

as infant cereals, to your infant's diet is one way to increase iron intake. Hummus and fortified tofu (shown below) are also good iron-rich foods that can be added from six months of age.

SUPPLEMENTS FOR BABIES

If you are following a strict plant-based diet with no animal products, you may need to consider supplements. The American Academy of Pediatrics recommends giving 400 IU a day of vitamin D to infants less than 1 year of age and 600 IU a day over 1 year. If you are weaning with mostly plant-based food, or if you are breastfeeding and vegan, you may need to consider further supplementation—talk with your doctor. Formula-fed babies may need less or different supplementation because formula is fortified with different vitamins and minerals.

When to wean

ALTHOUGH MOST BEGIN WEANING AT SIX MONTHS, ALL BABIES ARE DIFFERENT.

If you're unsure whether your child is ready, seek advice from a healthcare professional.
A baby is often ready to start eating food alongside milk when they show these key signs of readiness:

- Staying in a stable sitting position and holding their head steady.

- Swallowing the food given to them rather than spitting it back out.

- Coordinating their hands, eyes, and mouth so that when they look at food they pick it up and bring it toward their mouth.

Finger foods should be cut into sticks as they are easier for babies to grab in their palms. The texture should be soft enough to squish between forefinger and thumb.

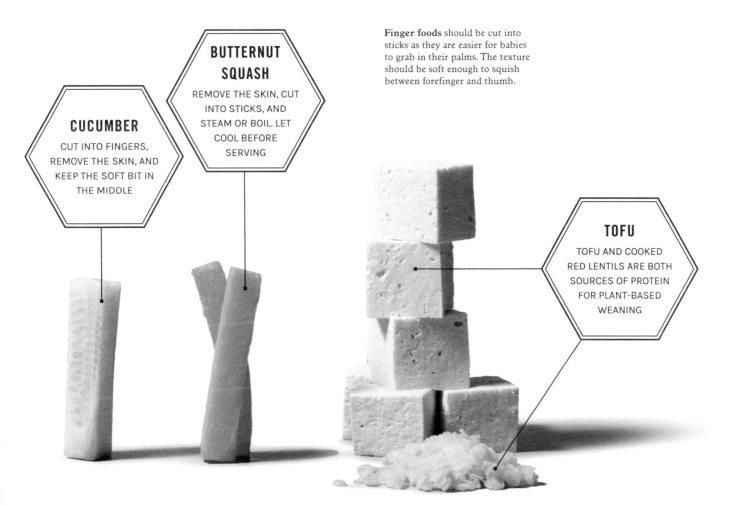

CUCUMBER
CUT INTO FINGERS, REMOVE THE SKIN, AND KEEP THE SOFT BIT IN THE MIDDLE

BUTTERNUT SQUASH
REMOVE THE SKIN, CUT INTO STICKS, AND STEAM OR BOIL. LET COOL BEFORE SERVING

TOFU
TOFU AND COOKED RED LENTILS ARE BOTH SOURCES OF PROTEIN FOR PLANT-BASED WEANING

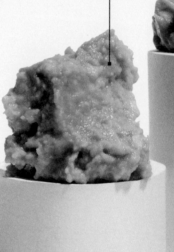

HUMMUS

THIS CHICKPEA-BASED DIP CONTAINS CALCIUM AND ARGININE, WHICH CAN BE LACKING IN A VEGAN DIET

AVOCADO

THESE FRUITS ARE AN ENERGY- AND NUTRIENT-DENSE SOURCE OF HEALTHY FATS AND ESSENTIAL AMINO ACIDS

NUT BUTTERS

ARE A GOOD SOURCE OF CONDITIONAL AMINO ACIDS, ENERGY, AND HEALTHY FATS

Nutrient-rich foods
Various nutrients may be lacking if feeding your baby a vegan or vegetarian diet. Supplements are the best option in many cases, but often those needs can be met by introducing certain nutrient-rich plant foods to your baby's diet, such as hummus, avocado, and nut butters.

SOURCES OF CONDITIONAL AMINO ACIDS

ARGININE	HISTIDINE	CYSTEINE	TYROSINE	GLUTAMINE	PROLINE
PUMPKIN SEEDS	TOFU	SUNFLOWER SEEDS	MILK	SOYBEANS	BEANS
SOYBEANS	PUMPKIN SEEDS	LENTILS	LENTILS	RED CABBAGE	NUTS
PEANUTS	WHOLE WHEAT PASTA	OATS	PUMPKIN SEEDS	NUTS	SEEDS
CHICKPEAS	HARICOT BEANS	CARROTS	WILD RICE	BEANS	
LENTILS					

CAN I RAISE MY CHILD VEGAN?

Veganism is becoming an increasingly popular choice for raising children for many reasons, including ethical and sustainability reasons. Existing research demonstrates that it is possible to feed your child a healthy and well-balanced vegan diet.

One study of almost 9,000 children aged six months to eight years reported no meaningful differences in the growth of those who were vegetarian compared to those who consumed meat in their diet. Other smaller studies have shown that vegan children are slightly lighter than meat-eaters but their weight is still within a healthy range. Vegan diets for babies and children require careful planning, and supplementation is recommended. Key areas to consider include nutrient density of the diet, protein intake, and appropriate sources of vitamins and minerals.

ENERGY INTAKES

Energy intake is an important and often overlooked aspect of childhood nutrition, and there is currently no public health calorie guideline set specifically for babies. Broadly, it is essential to provide sufficient calories, important healthy fats, and protein for infants and children to promote healthy growth and development. Vegan diets tend to have a higher fiber content, and too much fiber in the diet can fill up little tummies quickly. This means food quantity, energy, and nutrient intake from other sources may be reduced, which can lead to dietary deficiencies and a reduced energy intake. Make sure to include energy and nutrient-dense foods in the diet such as avocados, nuts (ground or butters), vegetable oils, seeds (ground or butters), tofu, pulses and legumes like lentils, soybeans, beans in general, chickpeas, and hummus. If there is a family history of allergy, consult a health professional before giving nut butter at 6 months. For vegetarian children, some

animal products such as full-fat dairy products and eggs may also be offered, which provide nutrient and energy-dense sources of protein and healthy fats.

PROTEIN

Protein is essential for your little one's growth, as well as for the maintenance and repair of their bodies. Protein requirements can be easily met if your child eats a wide variety of foods that contain protein at each meal. Beans, pulses, peas, lentils, nuts (again, if there is a family history of allergy, consult a health professional before giving nut butter at 6 months), grains such as quinoa, rice, buckwheat, and soy-based products like tofu are great sources of protein for your child. Conditional amino acids are usually considered nonessential as the body can make them on their own. Arginine is one example, and it can be missing in vegan diets.

IMPORTANT NUTRIENTS

Calcium, iron, omega-3, iodine, and vitamins A, C, and D are all important to consider for children on a vegan diet (see pp.166–167). Vitamin B12 is also often lacking in plant-based and vegan diets as many sources are animal-based (see pp.110–111). It is needed to support brain development and produce healthy red blood cells. Try to include foods that have been fortified with vitamin B12 in your child's daily diet, such as fortified unsweetened soy milk (do not offer as a drink until your child is 1 year old). If vegan, you may also need to supplement 5mcg a day up to 3 years old and 25mcg a day between 4 and 10 years old.

HOW CAN I AVOID NUTRIENT DEFICIENCIES IN BABIES AND YOUNG CHILDREN?

Making sure your little one eats nutritiously enables them to thrive in this period of rapid growth, development, and exploration. Adequate nutrition is important if we want to keep our bodies healthy and functioning optimally, and the most growth happens in the first 1,000 days.

———————

When we don't eat enough of the right foods or there is a lack of variety within the diet, it can lead to a deficiency in certain nutrients, particularly micronutrients. Nutrient deficiencies in children can include iron and vitamin D deficiencies, which may lead to conditions, including anemia, rickets, muscle aches and pains, deformities, and delayed growth and development. Deficiencies can have many negative and debilitating effects on the body, regardless of age, so it's important we optimize our own and our children's diets to ensure these are avoided.

FOOD ALLERGIES

An allergy occurs when the immune system reacts to a particular food and treats it as a threat, releasing chemicals that can result in serious symptoms. These include itching, feeling sick, vomiting, wheezing, and breathing problems. Research now suggests that early introduction of foods known to be allergens may help prevent allergies later in life and that introducing foods such as peanuts before six months of age may be beneficial.

Identifying and managing allergies is crucial, as they can lead to nutritional deficiencies. For instance, a dairy allergy may result in calcium and vitamin D deficiencies, impacting bone health. An egg allergy may contribute to a lack of essential proteins, and nut allergies can limit healthy fat intake, affecting brain development. To prevent deficiencies, you need to replace allergenic foods with suitable alternatives. To address calcium needs, children with dairy allergies can turn to fortified plant-based milk and yogurt. Substitutes for nut allergies include seeds and seed butters like tahini, while protein sources like tofu and legumes can replace eggs. Gluten avoidance may lead to insufficient intake of B vitamins and fiber. To counter this, incorporating gluten-free grains such as quinoa, rice, and gluten-free oats, along with a variety of fruits and vegetables, can provide necessary nutrients.

If you find that your child is experiencing challenges due to food allergies, it's important to speak with your healthcare provider for support and guidance on how best to manage it.

SMALLER STOMACHS

Young children and babies have very small stomachs. This means they need to eat more often than adults to get enough nutrients throughout the day. To help manage this, offer smaller portions of food, at more frequent intervals across the course of a day.

Too much fiber in the diet can quickly fill up the smaller digestive tract of a baby or young child, meaning food and nutrient intake from other sources may be reduced, leading to deficiencies.

VEGAN/VEGETARIAN/PLANT-BASED DIETS

Simply put, when raising your child as vegan, vegetarian, or plant-based, it is possible to give them all the nutrients they need for optimal growth and development. However, it requires careful planning, and it is likely you will need to supplement to ensure they are meeting nutritional requirements.

A NOTE OF CAUTION

Following a balanced, varied, and healthy diet is the best way to ensure your child is meeting all of their nutrient requirements. If, however, you think your child needs supplements, you should seek advice from your healthcare provider. It is possible to take too many vitamins, which can be detrimental to your health and that of your child.

Picky eating

PERSISTENT PICKY EATING, OR A LACK OF VARIETY WITHIN THE DIET—PARTICULARLY WITH FRUITS AND VEGETABLES, CAN INCREASE THE RISK OF VITAMIN AND MINERAL DEFICIENCIES. It may also mean that babies and children are not meeting the energy requirements to help support their growth and development. The key here is to be consistent and patient. Offer a variety of colors, textures, and flavors, as well as encourage good role modeling by eating a range of fruits and vegetables yourself and creating a positive and calming environment for your child to eat in.

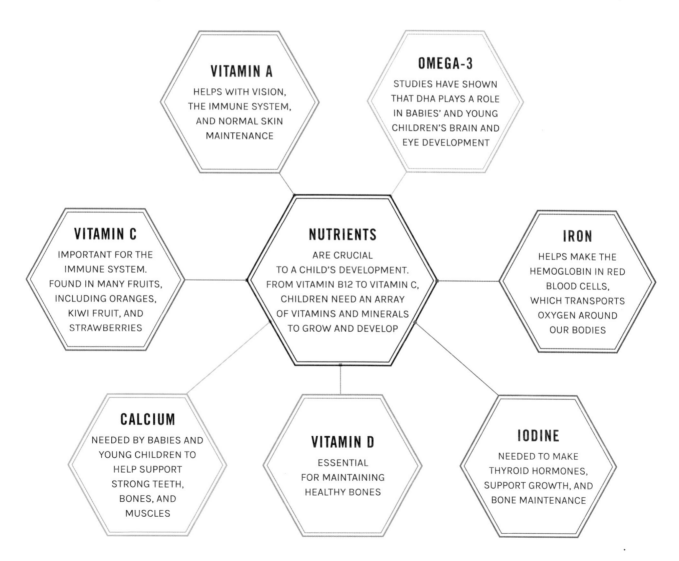

VITAMIN A
HELPS WITH VISION, THE IMMUNE SYSTEM, AND NORMAL SKIN MAINTENANCE

OMEGA-3
STUDIES HAVE SHOWN THAT DHA PLAYS A ROLE IN BABIES' AND YOUNG CHILDREN'S BRAIN AND EYE DEVELOPMENT

VITAMIN C
IMPORTANT FOR THE IMMUNE SYSTEM. FOUND IN MANY FRUITS, INCLUDING ORANGES, KIWI FRUIT, AND STRAWBERRIES

NUTRIENTS
ARE CRUCIAL TO A CHILD'S DEVELOPMENT. FROM VITAMIN B12 TO VITAMIN C, CHILDREN NEED AN ARRAY OF VITAMINS AND MINERALS TO GROW AND DEVELOP

IRON
HELPS MAKE THE HEMOGLOBIN IN RED BLOOD CELLS, WHICH TRANSPORTS OXYGEN AROUND OUR BODIES

CALCIUM
NEEDED BY BABIES AND YOUNG CHILDREN TO HELP SUPPORT STRONG TEETH, BONES, AND MUSCLES

VITAMIN D
ESSENTIAL FOR MAINTAINING HEALTHY BONES

IODINE
NEEDED TO MAKE THYROID HORMONES, SUPPORT GROWTH, AND BONE MAINTENANCE

WILL EATING PLANT-BASED HELP WITH MENOPAUSE?

Menopause can be a difficult time to navigate for many women, and a lack of research, support, and accessible information in recent times hasn't helped. Finally, steps are being taken to change this, but can our diet have an impact?

Diet can play a role in how we feel every day, and while there isn't a menopause diet that is rooted in evidence, there is some research to suggest that adherence to the Mediterranean diet (see p.37) is linked with reduced menopause symptoms.

PHYTOESTROGENS

Many plant-based foods contain phytoestrogens, which are believed to help with some of the symptoms of menopause, including hot flashes. These phytoestrogens bind with estrogen receptor sites in the body and act like naturally occurring estrogen. If you eat more plant-based foods, such as soy milk, flaxseed, tofu, tempeh, miso, and pumpkin seeds, this may help with your symptoms. Interestingly, in Asian countries where more of these foods are eaten, women are reported to experience fewer menopausal symptoms such as night sweats, vaginal dryness, and hot flushes than those in the US, although research is divided. Two servings of soy a day are recommended in order to get some of the benefits. Some people are able to produce an antioxidant compound called equol when they eat soy products, and there is some evidence to suggest that increased equol improves menopause symptoms.

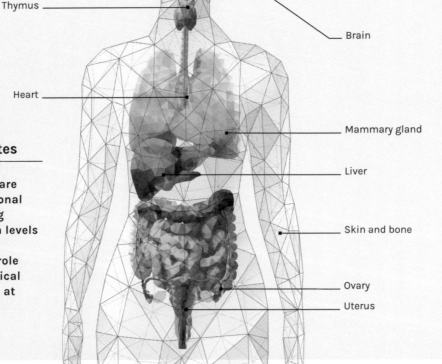

Thymus

Brain

Heart

Mammary gland

Liver

Skin and bone

Ovary

Uterus

Estrogen receptor sites

Estrogen receptor sites are key players in the hormonal shift experienced during menopause. As estrogen levels decline, these receptors around the body play a role in the diverse physiological changes that take place at this time.

GUT HEALTH

Good gut health is crucial for reducing our risk of disease and keeping us well, but it has also been linked to helping keep our estrogen levels balanced, which may help reduce menopausal symptoms. In one study of 17,000 menopausal women, those who consumed more fiber from vegetables and fruits and ate soy had a 19 percent reduction in hot flashes compared to the control group. Interestingly, the UK Women's Cohort Study of over 900 women showed that consuming a diet of foods beneficial for the gut, mostly plants such as pulses, fruits, and vegetables, which are high in prebiotic fiber for the gut microbes (see pp.16–17), could delay onset of the natural menopause by more than four years.

GROWING RESEARCH

Around the world, there is growing interest in diet and supporting the female aging process. One study found whole plant food intake was associated with reduced menopause symptoms. Furthermore, Chinese participants and a review of observational and many high-quality studies found that sticking to a Mediterranean diet can reduce negative health outcomes that are common after menopause, such as high cholesterol, low bone mineral density, and breast cancer risk.

A study in 2022 of diet and women of menopausal age had some interesting results. It showed that following a Mediterranean diet was associated with lower severity of menopausal symptoms in women with obesity. Consumption of legumes (beans, peas, and lentils) in particular was linked with less severe menopausal symptoms, and extra-virgin olive oil was associated with a reduction in psychological symptoms. These findings highlight the importance of this way of eating as an ideal nutritional strategy in the management of menopause.

Ultimately, while this area of research is lacking and we need more data to make any large conclusions, it looks like there is no harm in opting for a diet that contains whole foods that is essentially plant-based. Speak to your healthcare provider if you are suffering with menopause symptoms.

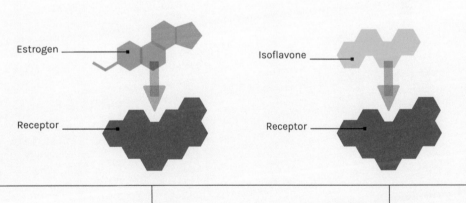

Estrogen

Receptor

Isoflavone

Receptor

Estrogen from soy

Phytoestrogens called isoflavones found in soy are structurally similar to human estrogen. They can bind to estrogen receptors in the body and mimic responses similar to those triggered by the body's own estrogen.

ESTROGEN

Human estrogen is able to bind to both types of estrogen receptors found on organs and tissues around the body.

PHYTOESTROGEN

Phytoestrogen, found in soy foods, binds to one type of estrogen receptor and may provide mild estrogen-like effects in some people.

CAN A PLANT-BASED DIET HELP WITH MENSTRUAL SYMPTOMS?

Period cramps, aches, and hormonal mood fluctuations can be tricky to manage, but more research is now emerging surrounding how what you eat can help with the symptoms of menstruation.

Research into women's health in the past has been lacking, but we are seeing more investment into the influence nutrition can have on the effects of premenstrual syndrome (PMS) and periods. We now know that certain foods can help relieve symptoms and are worth including in your daily diet.

PREMENSTRUAL SYNDROME

Premenstrual syndrome (PMS) is the term used for a group of symptoms that many experience in the week leading up to their period. These can include mood swings, headaches, acne, bloating, lower backache, fatigue, and breast tenderness, although not all women suffer all of these. Eating a Mediterranean diet (see p.37), which is largely plant-based, may help with premenstrual syndrome. Whole grain intake has been linked with reduced physical, mood, and behavioral symptoms associated with premenstrual syndrome. Making sure that you are consuming the right levels of calcium (see

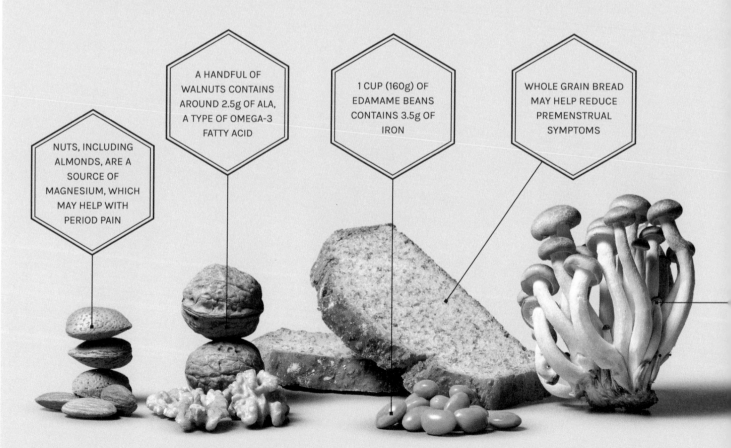

NUTS, INCLUDING ALMONDS, ARE A SOURCE OF MAGNESIUM, WHICH MAY HELP WITH PERIOD PAIN

A HANDFUL OF WALNUTS CONTAINS AROUND 2.5g OF ALA, A TYPE OF OMEGA-3 FATTY ACID

1 CUP (160g) OF EDAMAME BEANS CONTAINS 3.5g OF IRON

WHOLE GRAIN BREAD MAY HELP REDUCE PREMENSTRUAL SYMPTOMS

THE MENSTRUAL CYCLE

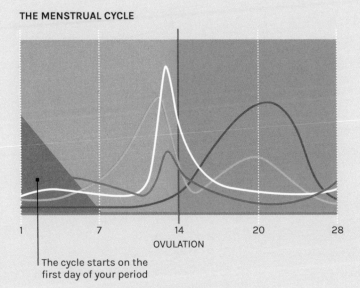

1   7   14   20   28

OVULATION

The cycle starts on the first day of your period

KEY

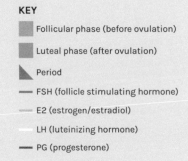

Follicular phase (before ovulation)

Luteal phase (after ovulation)

Period

FSH (follicle stimulating hormone)

E2 (estrogen/estradiol)

LH (luteinizing hormone)

PG (progesterone)

Phases of the menstrual cycle There are three phases in the cycle – follicular, ovulation, and luteal. Research suggests diet can play a role in the symptoms associated with these phases.

pp.100–101) and vitamin D (see pp.104–105), either through food or supplements, may help relieve some of these issues. Iron is also important to consider as the body loses iron in menstrual blood (see pp.98–99).

PERIOD PAIN

Cramps, also known as dysmenorrhea, affect most women during their period and are caused by inflammatory compounds called prostaglandins. These cause the uterine muscle to contract and release blood. Intake of magnesium and omega-3 may help reduce the intensity of the pain. Vitamins

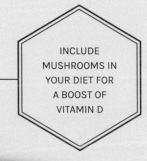

INCLUDE MUSHROOMS IN YOUR DIET FOR A BOOST OF VITAMIN D

Getting the right nutrients Eating a range of plant foods every week should improve your symptoms of PMS and period pain.

D and E are also believed to be beneficial, and ginger may help as it has some anti-inflammatory and analgesic effects.

Limited research suggests there is an association between plant-based diets and reduced menstrual symptoms, such as reduced bleeding. Lighter menstrual bleeding has also been associated with daily olive oil consumption, while the bleeding was heavier when eating ham on a weekly basis.

POLYCYSTIC OVARY SYNDROME AND ENDOMETRIOSIS

Small studies have shown that a plant-based diet may be helpful for those affected by polycystic ovary syndrome (PCOS). This is a hormonal disorder that causes irregular periods, an increase in the production of the male hormone androgen, and enlarged ovaries containing fluid-filled sacs called follicles. The condition can also lead to insulin resistance and type 2 diabetes. A low GI (glycemic index) diet, which is high in fruits, vegetables, and whole grains, can help reduce blood glucose levels and reduce the risk of diabetes developing. This kind of diet is easy to follow for plant-based eaters, although it's best to speak to your healthcare provider if you have the condition.

DOES PLANT-BASED EATING HELP CONTROL BLOOD SUGAR LEVELS?

Understanding how to manage our blood sugar levels can make the difference between feeling energized and ready for the day or feeling sluggish and lethargic. Simple changes to your diet can help you avoid these problems.

By blood sugar levels, we mean how much glucose from the food we eat is in our blood at any one time. We get glucose from foods containing carbohydrates, and the average adult requires 200g of carbs per day. Ensuring our glucose stores don't dip too low can enhance our performance, mood, and daily bodily functions.

THE BLOOD SUGAR ROLLER COASTER

Your blood sugar levels go up and down naturally throughout the day, but to ensure they don't fluctuate too drastically, you can manipulate your diet to ease the blood sugar roller coaster. To do this, you need to understand how the body processes blood sugar. Our bodies have a very effective system in place to handle a rise in glucose when we eat—the pancreas releases insulin to help the uptake of glucose into our cells and removes it from our bloodstream. Our liver and muscles take glucose and use it for immediate energy or store as glycogen. Those with a lack of insulin, or an inability to adequately respond to insulin, can develop diabetes.

New research is showing that blood sugar reactions to food vary between people. Growing

Blood sugar highs and lows

When you eat a lot of refined carbs, your pancreas sees a spike in blood glucose levels and releases insulin as quickly as it can to try to catch up. This can result in too much glucose being removed from your blood, causing a blood sugar crash that can leave you feeling fatigued, irritable, depressed, anxious, and nervous.

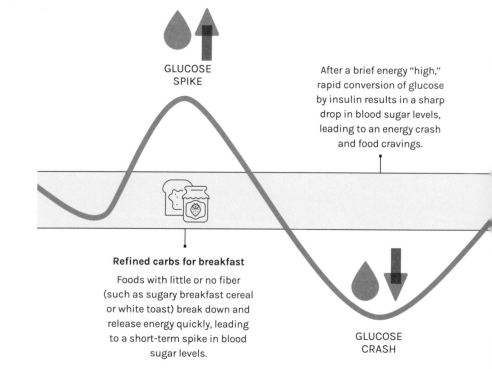

GLUCOSE SPIKE

After a brief energy "high," rapid conversion of glucose by insulin results in a sharp drop in blood sugar levels, leading to an energy crash and food cravings.

Refined carbs for breakfast
Foods with little or no fiber (such as sugary breakfast cereal or white toast) break down and release energy quickly, leading to a short-term spike in blood sugar levels.

GLUCOSE CRASH

numbers, not just those with diabetes, are now using personalized blood sugar monitors to keep track of their blood sugar levels continuously. These help you can see how diet, exercise, sleep, and stress affects your blood sugar.

DIET AND BLOOD SUGAR

The type of food we eat can impact the duration of this process and how the peaks and troughs in our blood sugar levels are formed throughout the day. The difference between sugar, refined carbohydrates, and whole foods is how long this conversion takes. Foods with lots of fiber (whole grains and vegetables) take longer; foods with less or no fiber (white carbs and sugar) digest much more quickly. Plant-based diets are often mistakenly thought of as being terrible for our blood sugar balance because they are "high in carbs," but there is a lack of understanding on fiber content, vegetarian protein sources, fats, and whole foods involved.

A well-planned plant-based diet may be more beneficial for blood sugar levels than a poorly executed animal protein diet. Studies have found that after adopting a vegetarian or vegan diet, glycemic control often improves, and in many cases, patients can decrease or discontinue their type 2 diabetes medication (always consult your doctor).

Plant-based diets can potentially lead to weight loss (see pp.196–197), especially visceral fat which builds up around the internal organs, and this improves insulin sensitivity. In addition, plant diets are often rich in soluble fiber, which slows glucose absorption. Some plant proteins like soy also contain carbohydrates that provide amino acids and micronutrients that can improve insulin sensitivity and glycemic control. In a study of nearly 3,000 Buddhists, those with a lifelong adherence to a vegetarian diet had a 35 percent lower risk of developing type 2 diabetes, indicating healthy blood sugar balance.

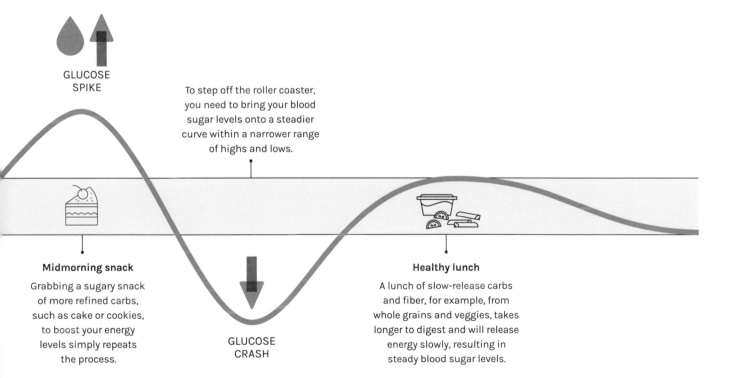

GLUCOSE SPIKE

To step off the roller coaster, you need to bring your blood sugar levels onto a steadier curve within a narrower range of highs and lows.

GLUCOSE CRASH

Midmorning snack

Grabbing a sugary snack of more refined carbs, such as cake or cookies, to boost your energy levels simply repeats the process.

Healthy lunch

A lunch of slow-release carbs and fiber, for example, from whole grains and veggies, takes longer to digest and will release energy slowly, resulting in steady blood sugar levels.

CAN I BE A
PLANT-BASED ATHLETE?

With the increased visibility of high-profile vegan athletes, such as Venus Williams and Lewis Hamilton, it is entirely possible to be a plant-based athlete, but you need to plan carefully to ensure you eat correctly for your sport.

While some people may remain skeptical, it has been proven for a long time that you don't need to consume animal products to perform well and at the highest levels. First, understanding that sports nutrition is different from public health nutrition is key; sports nutrition is methodical, calculated, and used as a tool to optimize performance. As long as an athlete achieves their macronutrient intake and micronutrient intake, with some supplementation where necessary, there are no negatives to consuming a plant-based diet. Research has shown that there is no difference in performance between those consuming a plant-based diet and those eating a diet containing meat and dairy foods. No differences in strength, anaerobic, or aerobic performance have been identified.

KEY SPORTS NUTRITION COMPONENTS

A plant-based diet contains all of the key areas of sports nutrition required. Energy density may need to be addressed, though, as generally there are fewer calories in large portions of plant whole foods than in animal products. Choosing balanced meals carefully, with supplements if required, will enable a high-level performance and also aid a speedy and effective recovery following sports activities.

● **Carbohydrates** These are important to fuel any form of exercise, but the amount you require depends on the duration of the sport and its intensity. Carbohydrate intake is especially important for athletes as it provides the readiest form of energy. It is needed for short bursts of high-intensity training.

● **Protein** It is important to ensure we consume enough of this macronutrient for daily functions and

KEY

▬ Glycogen/glucose

▬ Fat

Fat vs. glycogen use While actual usage depends on the intensity at which you do any exercise, and individual fitness levels, broadly speaking, some activities burn more fuel from fat stores than glycogen in muscles.

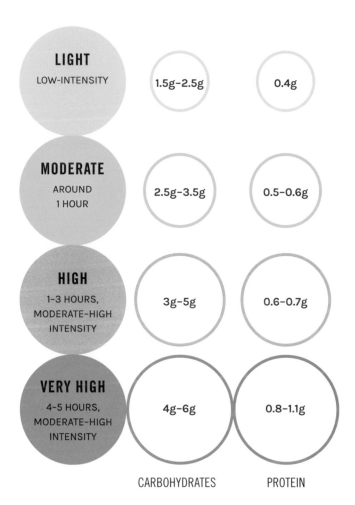

LIGHT
LOW-INTENSITY

1.5g–2.5g

0.4g

MODERATE
AROUND
1 HOUR

2.5g–3.5g

0.5–0.6g

HIGH
1–3 HOURS,
MODERATE–HIGH
INTENSITY

3g–5g

0.6–0.7g

VERY HIGH
4–5 HOURS,
MODERATE–HIGH
INTENSITY

4g–6g

0.8–1.1g

CARBOHYDRATES

PROTEIN

Macronutrient requirements Your daily needs measured in grams by pound of body weight, based on your individual activity level. For example, someone weighing 165lb (75kg) who engages in a high volume of exercise will require 4–6g of carbohydrates for every pound body weight. Unlike carbs and protein, there are no specific official recommendations for fat intake. Active individuals and athletes should follow government guidelines.

more if working toward athletic goals and muscle building. If we do not consume enough energy from carbohydrates, our body may use protein for fuel, which means that it can't be used to build or maintain muscle mass. As protein is more effectively absorbed from food than from supplements (although there is good research supporting the efficacy of whey protein), it is crucial to maximize dietary variety and intake throughout the day. Good sources of plant protein include beans, pulses, yogurts, nuts, seeds, tofu, and meat alternatives like Quorn. A variety is important because not every plant protein contains all of the key amino acids, so by eating a variety of protein sources, you are less likely to fall short.

● **Fat** is used as a fuel when our glycogen stores run low. At least 20 percent of your overall calorie intake should come from fats.
● **Hydration** Fluid intake is important to ensure your heart works efficiently. Fluid and sodium loss can impact your performance by up to 20 percent. You may feel tired, which can make exercise harder. Dehydration and fluid loss of more than 2–3 percent of your body weight can impair performance.
● **Supplements** There is evidence supporting some sports supplements for enhancing performance. They may be useful, if required, for those eating a plant-based diet to make sure they are getting the additional vitamins and minerals required (see pp.96–97).

WILL PLANT-BASED NUTRITION HELP ME SLEEP?

Sleep is a basic human necessity, but one in three adults is not getting enough, and up to 70 million Americans have chronic sleep disorders. Emerging research suggests our diets may play a larger role than previously thought.

Not getting enough sleep can have a lot of negative consequences for our daily lives at work or school, while driving, and functioning in a social capacity. Difficulties can occur with learning, focusing, and reacting. Also, you might find it hard to judge other people's emotions and reactions, leaving you feeling frustrated, irritable, or anxious in social situations. More worryingly, there is a link between sleep deficiency and chronic health problems, including heart disease, kidney disease, high blood pressure, diabetes, stroke, obesity, and depression.

DIET AND SLEEP

It is generally known that lifestyle factors such as stress and exercise contribute to quality sleep, but improving your diet may also help. Nutrition can influence the quality of your sleep, and some foods and drinks can make it easier or harder to get the sleep that you need. It is difficult to establish the cause and effect, but we know that diet plays a role in the hormones involved in the process of sleep. Plant-based diets hold the key components needed to help contribute to a good night's sleep, with vegetables and fruits helping provide the vitamins and minerals we need to function well. One study reported that those deficient in nutrients such as calcium, magnesium, and vitamins A, C, D, E, and K

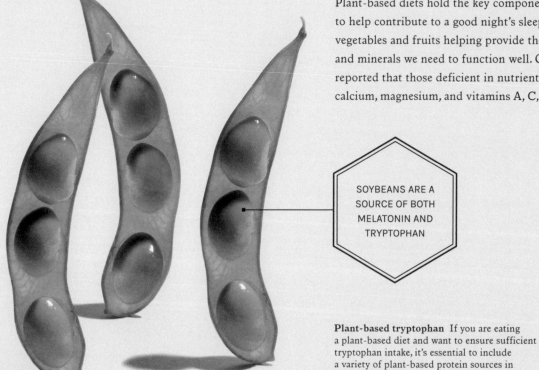

SOYBEANS ARE A SOURCE OF BOTH MELATONIN AND TRYPTOPHAN

Plant-based tryptophan If you are eating a plant-based diet and want to ensure sufficient tryptophan intake, it's essential to include a variety of plant-based protein sources in your meals.

TRYPTOPHAN

THE ESSENTIAL AMINO ACID IS OBTAINED FROM FOODS INCLUDING GRAINS, SEEDS, AND LEGUMES

5-HTP

TRYPTOPHAN IS CONVERTED INTO A COMPOUND CALLED 5-HYDROXYTRYPTOPHAN (5-HTP)

SEROTONIN

5-HTP IS CONVERTED INTO SEROTONIN, WHICH HELPS WITH MOOD REGULATION

MELATONIN

SEROTONIN IS CONVERTED INTO MELATONIN. LEVELS RISE IN THE EVENING AS WE PREPARE FOR SLEEP

Tryptophan conversion to melatonin The essential amino acid is the precursor to melatonin, which is known to help sleep.

had more sleep problems than other people. Other micronutrients that may improve sleep are vitamin B1 (thiamine), B9 (folate), phosphorus, iron, zinc, and selenium.

BLOOD SUGAR

You may have heard that carbohydrates make you drowsy, and there is some truth to this, as they can affect blood sugar levels and insulin (see pp.172–173), directly affecting our energy levels. Eating carbs can lead to a spike in blood sugar levels followed by a drop, leaving you feeling tired. It is not recommended that you eat carbs in order to help you sleep as this can potentially lead to the development of diabetes. Avoid energy drinks and sugar-sweetened beverages as they raise blood sugar levels, which can affect sleep patterns.

AVOID STIMULANTS

Alcohol and being overweight may enhance the risk of developing serious sleep conditions, such as obstructive sleep apnea (OSA), a condition where obstructions in the airway can cause a range of issues. Most people are aware that caffeine is a stimulant that affects sleep, but so does theobromine, which is consumed in cocoa and chocolate beverages and in various forms of chocolate-based foods. These work by blocking adenosine (which promotes the drive to sleep) providing energy immediately after consumption but having long-lasting consequences that can alter sleep patterns for hours after eating. These consequences include prolonged sleep latency (taking a long time to fall asleep), reduced total sleep time, sleep inefficiency (the amount of time you spend asleep in bed versus time spent in bed), poor sleep quality, and REM sleep behavior disorder, which involves the person

having vivid and intense dreams and moving, kicking, and punching during sleep.

HORMONES AND SLEEP

Melatonin is a hormone produced in the pineal gland of the brain when we are in a dark environment and is believed to help us sleep better. Certain foods contain melatonin and eating more of them could help. Foods containing the amino acid tryptophan are also important because tryptophan can be converted into serotonin and then into melatonin in the body. Due to its role in the production of serotonin (known as a natural mood stabilizer), tryptophan is sometimes given as a supplement to reduce depression, although this is not usually necessary if you're eating a healthy, balanced diet.

DO FOODS CONTAIN MELATONIN?

The term phytomelatonin refers to melatonin from plants and algae and is widely used to differentiate it from animal and/or synthetic melatonin. Research on the bioavailability of dietary melatonin is still quite scarce. This may be because measuring the bioavailability requires serum samples (the liquid component of blood). Also this area of research is complex because readings of melatonin levels can be masked by other vitamins and minerals consumed at the same time. Additionally, levels of melatonin in plants differ widely, even within the same species, so bioavailability cannot be assured.

For individuals following a plant-based diet who are concerned about their melatonin intake, focus on factors that support the body's natural melatonin production. These include maintaining a consistent sleep schedule, creating a sleep-friendly environment, and managing stress.

COULD A PLANT-BASED DIET SUPPORT MY MENTAL HEALTH?

Mental health impacts everyone; it does not discriminate. According to the World Health Organization, in 2019, 970 million people around the world were living with a mental disorder, with anxiety and depressive disorders being the most common. The latest research suggests diet can influence our mood and mental health.

As mental health is discussed more widely, research is being done into diet and its impact on mood. Food is now being hailed as potentially more powerful in this area than some medication.

SEROTONIN AND HAPPINESS

The brain uses the amino acid tryptophan to produce serotonin, a neurotransmitter linked to feelings of happiness and wellness. Plant-based sources of tryptophan include leafy greens, sunflower seeds, watercress, soybeans, pumpkin seeds, mushrooms, broccoli, and peas. While meat such as turkey also contains this amino acid, the body can have a difficult time converting it to serotonin. This is because there is competition from other amino acids found in protein that prevent tryptophan from entering the brain. This can lead to low serotonin production. Adding more carbohydrates at each meal may promote an increase in insulin production, allowing muscle cells to absorb competing amino acids. This makes it easier for tryptophan to cross the blood-brain barrier, increasing serotonin levels.

OMEGA-3

Research has shown links between omega-3 fatty acids (see pp.102–103) and mental health. They are believed to assist in the release and transmission of serotonin and dopamine, which help regulate mood. Chronic brain inflammation is linked to mood disorders, and omega-3 has anti-inflammatory properties so may help with this.

REDUCE MEAT AND JUNK FOOD

There is support in the scientific world for reducing animal consumption as it is believed that there are links between arachidonic acid (a polyunsaturated omega-6 fatty acid found in eggs and meat) and depression. Junk food is also advised against as it contains additives and preservatives that can affect how you feel and behave. The refined sugars and carbs included may also cause fluctuations in blood sugar, linked to irritability and fatigue.

RESEARCH

Trials in 2017 showed some promising results around food and mood. They were the first of their kind to investigate the question "If I improve my diet, will my mood improve?" Over a 12-week trial, 67 participants with clinical depression were randomly assigned to one of two groups. One group focused on a Mediterranean diet (see p.37), and others were offered social support. The results were significant with 30 percent achieving full remission from depression in the diet group and just 8 percent recovering in the social support group. These findings may help us find new ways of treating depression.

The gut—brain axis

There is a link between the health of the gut and the brain. Neural pathways connect the brain to the gut. The brain influences intestinal microbiota, and the intestinal microbiota influence brain and behavior.

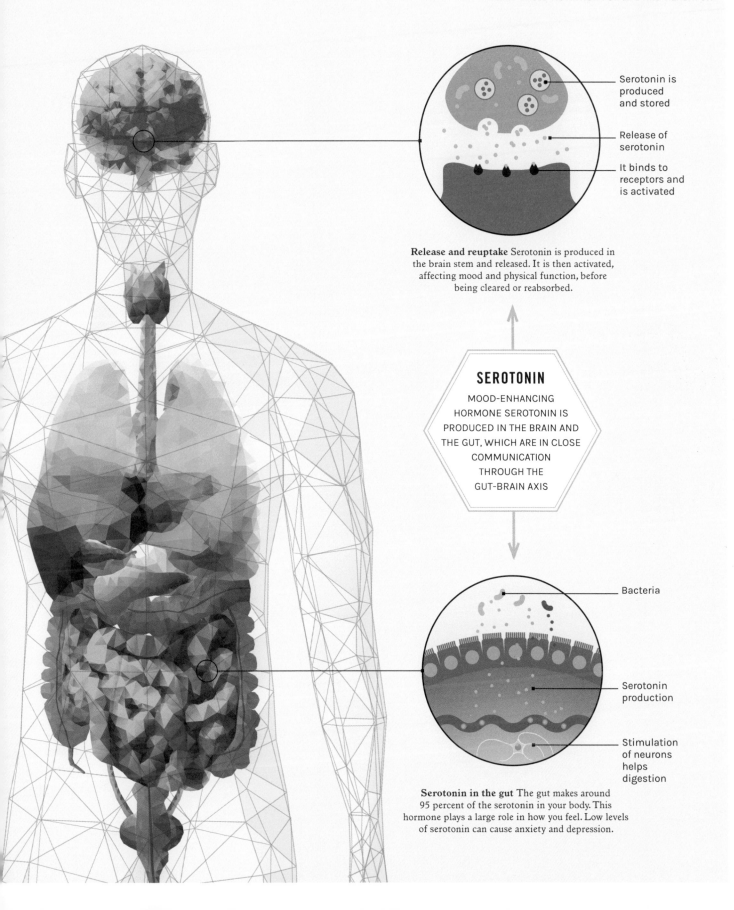

Serotonin is produced and stored

Release of serotonin

It binds to receptors and is activated

Release and reuptake Serotonin is produced in the brain stem and released. It is then activated, affecting mood and physical function, before being cleared or reabsorbed.

SEROTONIN

MOOD-ENHANCING HORMONE SEROTONIN IS PRODUCED IN THE BRAIN AND THE GUT, WHICH ARE IN CLOSE COMMUNICATION THROUGH THE GUT-BRAIN AXIS

Bacteria

Serotonin production

Stimulation of neurons helps digestion

Serotonin in the gut The gut makes around 95 percent of the serotonin in your body. This hormone plays a large role in how you feel. Low levels of serotonin can cause anxiety and depression.

DOES PLANT-BASED EATING IMPACT MALE HEALTH OUTCOMES?

According to recent figures, in the US, 79 percent of vegans identify as female . This is a pattern that is replicated in th UK with twice as many women claiming to be vegan than men. Should more men be thinking about eating a plant-based diet to benefit their health?

In a culture where the media around dieting is often gendered as a female concern and which categorizes meat as a "male" food choice, there is a theory that suggests there is an increased amount of pressure on women to change the way they eat and for men to follow the gender stereotypes. These behaviors are changing as younger generations of men and boys are more concerned with their appearance.

DEPRESSION

There hasn't been much research into the long-term health of men who eat a plant-based diet. That being said, however, one groundbreaking trial into plant-based diets and mental health included males and discovered that the diet was successful in managing clinical depression with reduced symptoms, although more research needs to be done in this area (see pp.178–179).

HEART DISEASE

The leading cause of death for men in many Western countries is heart disease. The most helpful diets for those looking at heart health are those with more fiber and less saturated fats, such as the Mediterranean diet. Adhering to this diet has also shown improvements in better quality and quantity of sleep for some men in small scale studies, which, in turn, can translate into better overall health.

CANCER

In men under 65 years of age diagnosed with prostate cancer, greater overall consumption of plant-based foods has been associated with a lower risk of advanced prostate cancer. Among younger men, greater consumption of a healthful plant-based diet has been associated with lower risks of prostate cancer. There is also some evidence to suggest that colon cancer could also be reduced by eating more plant-based foods. A large study that involved 79,952 US-based men found that those who ate the largest amounts of healthy plant-based foods had lower risk of colon cancer compared with those who ate the least.

There are many reasons plant-based diets may be helpful, including the antioxidant content in fruits and vegetables and potentially the fiber and links with gut health. Ultimately, men could benefit from consuming a healthy well-balanced plant-based diet, but we need more research in this area.

The benefits of plant-based eating

Eating plenty of heart-healthy foods like fruits and vegetables can help with male fertility.

FERTILITY

Another area where diet can have an effect is fertility. Research suggests that a well-balanced vegan diet can positively impact male fertility. Plant-based diets rich in fruits, vegetables, and whole grains contribute to overall health, which can indirectly influence reproductive function. Antioxidants found in plant-based foods may help combat oxidative stress, which can improve sperm count, quality, and motility.

LIBIDO

Consuming a plant-based diet with a variety of fruits, vegetables, whole grains, nuts, and seeds can positively influence factors that contribute to sexual well-being. A diet low in saturated fats and high in plant-based whole foods helps keep our hearts healthy. A healthy cardiovascular system is crucial for blood flow, which can impact sexual function and libido.

THE GENDER DIVIDE

Statistics show that among Western societies, women are twice as likely to follow a plant-based diet than men. Vegetarianism is falsely viewed as a stereotypically feminine behavior. In some sectors, vegetarian eating is seen as healthy, and healthful foods are seen as feminine, whereas eating less healthy foods is seen as masculine. Several factors contribute to this gender divide. Societal norms and cultural expectations can give the idea that masculinity is associated with meat consumption and that this makes men strong. Surveys and interviews have found that some men feel peer pressure to eat meat so that they appear more masculine. Women are also generally more health-conscious than men, which may lead them to follow a plant-based diet.

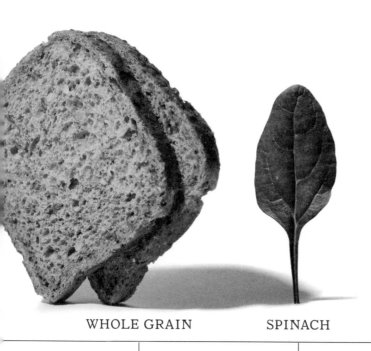

WHOLE GRAIN

Foods including whole grain bread, brown rice, and quinoa can support male reproductive health.

SPINACH

Dark leafy greens are good sources of vitamin B9 (folate), which is essential for sperm production.

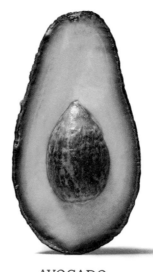
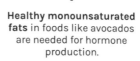

AVOCADO

Healthy monounsaturated fats in foods like avocados are needed for hormone production.

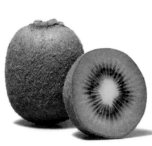

KIWI

Kiwi fruits are rich in vitamin C, an antioxidant that can support sperm health.

CAN A PLANT-BASED DIET SUPPORT THE AGING PROCESS?

Aging is embraced and seen as a privilege in some cultures, but by others, it is seen as a process to be delayed as long as possible. Good nutrition can help us stay well for longer as we grow older.

Improved social, medical, economic, and environmental hygiene conditions have led to a population explosion over the course of little more than a century. Over-65-year-olds are now the fastest growing age group globally, and over two billion people are predicted to be over 60 years old by 2050. This is good news as long as we can stay healthy as we age—our diet can play a huge role in this.

THE AGING PROCESS

Aging is a natural process in which cellular and molecular damage that takes place over time leads to a greater risk of age-related disorders. We cannot control the decline of health as we age, but we can enhance our quality of life through lifestyle and diet. Research suggests that changes in diet are crucial to prevent the emergence of disease, boost longevity, and promote healthy aging.

Many studies have explored the links between extra-virgin olive oil or nuts and the impact on cognitive function and neurodegenerative diseases such as Alzheimer's. The Mediterranean diet (see p.37), which includes high consumption of extra-virgin olive oil, is linked with reduced inflammation and frailty, and improved gut microbiome modulation, which may be a driving factor of healthy aging.

How excess sugar ages skin

Collagen and elastin keep skin firm but can be damaged by glycation. This process is accelerated by eating a lot of high GI (glycemic index) food, especially sugary foods, that rapidly convert to sugar in the blood.

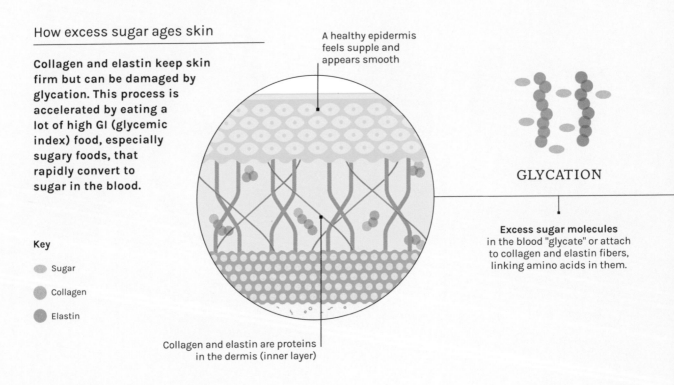

A healthy epidermis feels supple and appears smooth

GLYCATION

Excess sugar molecules in the blood "glycate" or attach to collagen and elastin fibers, linking amino acids in them.

Collagen and elastin are proteins in the dermis (inner layer)

Key

Sugar

Collagen

Elastin

AGE AND NUTRITION

Ensuring you are consuming adequate nutrition as you grow older is vital to support your bones, joints, cognition, and much more. The amount of nutrients your body absorbs can change over time. Some factors that particularly affect dietary intake in later years are sensory impairment (for example, loss of vision and taste), poor oral health, loss of mobility, and psychosocial changes, including poor finances and increased isolation. As we age, our gastric acid secretion also decreases, which can impact nutrient absorption. Gastric acid is crucial in the digestion of proteins and minerals and for vitamin B12 absorption. If we have less gastric acid, we may not be getting the maximum amount of nutrition from the food we consume. Here are some ways to stay as healthy as possible through diet:

● Avoid vitamin and mineral deficiencies—these are often linked to cognitive and physical decline. Eating a healthy Mediterranean-style diet containing fruits, vegetables, and protein and incorporating polyunsaturated fatty acids, with a focus on nutrient-dense foods, will ensure you get the nutrients you need. Vitamins D (see pp.104–105), C, and B9 impact our bones and inflammation. Vitamin B12 (see pp.110–111) is important for bone and neurological health and can be found in fortified foods such as plant-based milks.

● Calcium from leafy greens; zinc and iron from lentils, chickpeas, and seeds; and selenium found in Brazil nuts are important as they contribute to bone density and the immune system.

● Get enough protein from plant sources such as tofu and soybeans—this is important for muscle mass, and we may need more as we age.

● Ensure you include healthy unsaturated fats in your diet, particularly from extra-virgin olive oil, nuts, and seeds.

● Avoid foods and drinks containing added sugar, which damages your skin.

● Stay hydrated (see pp.24–25).

If you think you are not getting the right vitamins and minerals and need supplementation (see pp.96–97), seek the advice of your healthcare professional.

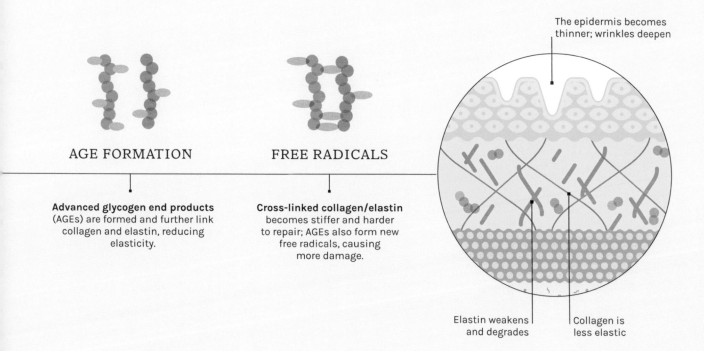

AGE FORMATION

FREE RADICALS

Advanced glycogen end products (AGEs) are formed and further link collagen and elastin, reducing elasticity.

Cross-linked collagen/elastin becomes stiffer and harder to repair; AGEs also form new free radicals, causing more damage.

The epidermis becomes thinner; wrinkles deepen

Elastin weakens and degrades

Collagen is less elastic

CAN PLANT-BASED NUTRITION SUPPORT YOUR IMMUNITY?

Nutrition plays a key role in supporting our immune system. As 70 percent of our immune system resides in our guts, it makes sense that we need to eat a healthy balanced diet to support this process.

———————

Your immune system is a network of cells, tissues, and organs that work to defend your body from harmful pathogens. It needs energy to fuel new immune cells to fight the threat, and your diet is important in this process. Claims that it is possible to boost your immune system by eating certain foods are false. Although you can support your immune system through diet, you cannot, and would not want to, boost it because an overactive immune system can lead to immune conditions. The best way to support your immune system is to eat a healthy diet. Your gut health and antibiotic use can also affect your immune response. Other factors, such as sleep and reducing stress levels, are important, but if you consider these factors and eat well, you will be supporting your health now and in the future. You should, however, plan out your diet and avoid any micronutrient deficiencies that can lead to a weakened immune system.

GUT MICROBES

The microbes that reside in our gut are in continuous communication with our immune cells (see pp.68–69) and train our immune system from the moment we are born. In order to ensure we support those gut microbes to do their job, we need to eat a balanced diet with a variety of plant foods. Eating 30 different plant types a week has been shown to provide us with flavonoids and fiber, which may help lower levels of inflammation (see pp.70–71).

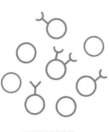

WHITE BLOOD CELLS

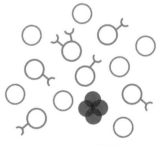

PATHOGEN DETECTED

The immune response

Two key immune responses work together. The natural response quickly tries to stop the pathogen spreading, while the slower adaptive response requires exposure to the pathogen first, then learns to identify it rapidly.

Different types of white blood cells patrol or wait to be alerted. Many types play a role in both stages of the immune response.

One/more of these cell types detect a pathogen via its antigen (surface protein). They multiply and signal other immune cells.

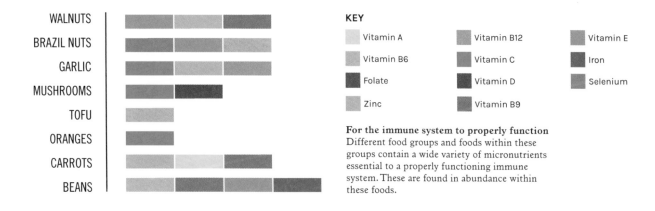

WALNUTS
BRAZIL NUTS
GARLIC
MUSHROOMS
TOFU
ORANGES
CARROTS
BEANS

KEY

Vitamin A

Vitamin B6

Folate

Zinc

Vitamin B12

Vitamin C

Vitamin D

Vitamin B9

Vitamin E

Iron

Selenium

For the immune system to properly function
Different food groups and foods within these groups contain a wide variety of micronutrients essential to a properly functioning immune system. These are found in abundance within these foods.

Plant-based diets that are higher in fiber help feed the short-chain fatty acids, which have been shown to improve immunity against pathogens.

PROBIOTICS AND PREBIOTICS

The majority of research suggests a well-balanced and varied plant-based diet is the best way of obtaining all the essential immune-supporting nutrients like vitamins B6 and D. Including probiotic foods into this diet is also beneficial, and although it includes dairy, dietitians and other clinical researchers have found that a probiotic milk drink containing *Lactobacillus casei* and *Lactobacillus bulgaricus* may prevent older people who are taking antibiotics in hospital from getting a superbug called C-diff. Prebiotics from plants are also helpful because they act as a fertilizer for our gut microbes, helping them flourish and do their job well (see pp.76–77). Plant-based diets tend to include more prebiotic foods than meat-based diets. In fact, one study showed that those following a low-carb or high-protein diet had close to four times the chance of becoming unwell with COVID-19, compared to those eating plant-based.

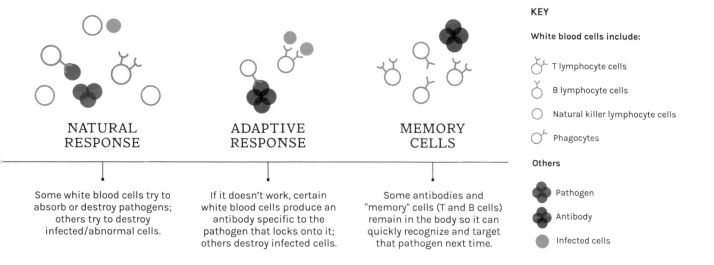

NATURAL RESPONSE

Some white blood cells try to absorb or destroy pathogens; others try to destroy infected/abnormal cells.

ADAPTIVE RESPONSE

If it doesn't work, certain white blood cells produce an antibody specific to the pathogen that locks onto it; others destroy infected cells.

MEMORY CELLS

Some antibodies and "memory" cells (T and B cells) remain in the body so it can quickly recognize and target that pathogen next time.

KEY

White blood cells include:

T lymphocyte cells

B lymphocyte cells

Natural killer lymphocyte cells

Phagocytes

Others

Pathogen

Antibody

Infected cells

IS PLANT-BASED NUTRITION BETTER FOR YOUR BONES?

If you are eating a plant-based diet you need to be aware of the key nutrients that keep your bones healthy and strong. Beyond diet, lifestyle factors, including physical activity and healthy body weight, play a role in bone health.

———————

Plant-based diets are not categorically better for bone health but can equate to the same support as diets that include meat and dairy if we ensure we are getting enough of the key nutrients required. We need to take care of our bones to avoid developing osteoporosis (see p.101). Due to its prevalence worldwide, osteoporosis is considered a serious public health concern, with 75 million people in Europe, the US, and Japan being affected by the condition.

CALCIUM AND VITAMIN D
Calcium is crucial for bone health, and vitamin D is needed to help your body absorb the calcium. Some important plant sources of calcium are fortified plant milks, tofu, and leafy green vegetables. An ideal calcium intake for adults is 1,000–1,200mg per day (see pp.100–101), but this may not be enough if you already have reduced bone mass density. If you are plant-based and find it hard to make up this amount from diet alone, you should take a daily calcium supplement providing 400–600mg of calcium, preferably alongside 400 IU of vitamin D. Adults aged 19 to 50 should not have more than 2,500mg calcium total per day (including food and supplements), and those over 50 should not exceed 2,000mg total per day. If you are unsure, speak to your healthcare provider who can advise you on which supplement to take. Calcium is considered safe, but too much in the form of supplements may increase the risk of kidney stones, constipation, or calcium buildup in your blood vessels and affect your ability to absorb iron and zinc.

VITAMIN K
Vitamin K is another essential nutrient for bone health. Most plant-based eaters will be getting enough if they have a variety of vegetables and fruits in the diet. Vitamin K1 is found in Brussels sprouts, cabbage, kale, broccoli, spinach, spring greens, spring onions, and kiwi fruit.

LOW WEIGHT
Generally, you are more likely to break a bone if your body mass index (BMI) is low because there is less cushioning around your hips and you may have less bone tissue. Ensure the plant-based diet you follow contains enough energy and include plenty of nutrient-dense foods such as nuts, seeds, and oils.

Remember antinutrients

PLANT FOODS MAY CONTAIN COMPOUNDS THAT REDUCE THE AMOUNT OF CALCIUM YOUR BODY CAN ABSORB.

Leafy green vegetables, like cooked broccoli, Brussels sprouts, kale, and collard greens, are sources of calcium. Calcium can also be found in beans and fortified plant milks. Remember, spinach, dried fruits, beans, seeds, and nuts may contain calcium, but they also contain oxalates and/or phytates, which reduce how much calcium your body can absorb from them. You should not rely on these foods as your main source of calcium.

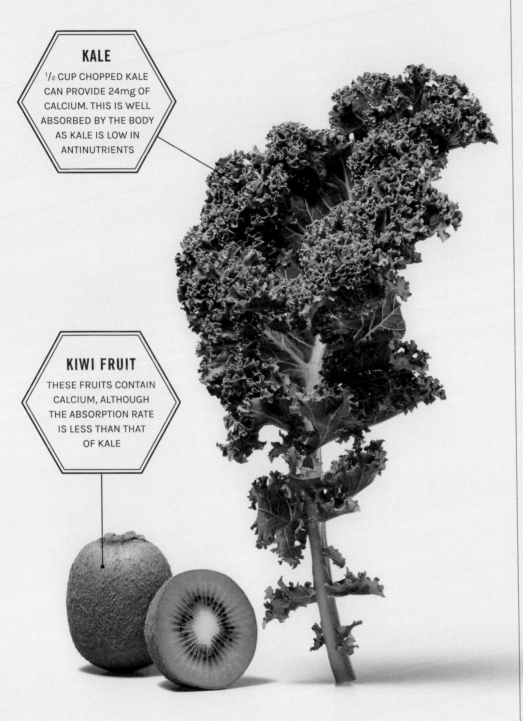

KALE

¹/₂ CUP CHOPPED KALE CAN PROVIDE 24mg OF CALCIUM. THIS IS WELL ABSORBED BY THE BODY AS KALE IS LOW IN ANTINUTRIENTS

KIWI FRUIT

THESE FRUITS CONTAIN CALCIUM, ALTHOUGH THE ABSORPTION RATE IS LESS THAN THAT OF KALE

Plant sources Both kale and kiwi fruits can provide bone-friendly calcium and vitamin K.

Other factors that impact bone health

APART FROM EATING A GOOD DIET, BE AWARE OF THE FOLLOWING:

LOW ESTROGEN

ESTROGEN REGULATES BONE METABOLISM. IT IS ESSENTIAL TO BONE HEALTH BECAUSE IT PROMOTES THE ACTIVITY OF CELLS THAT MAKE NEW BONE

WEIGHT

LOW BODY WEIGHT IS LINKED WITH LOW BONE MASS AND A HIGHER RISK OF FRACTURES

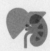

OTHER HEALTH CONDITIONS

MEDICAL CONDITIONS LIKE RHEUMATOID ARTHRITIS, CHRONIC KIDNEY DISEASE, OVERACTIVE PARATHYROID GLAND, AND SOME KINDS OF CANCER

LIFESTYLE FACTORS

SMOKING, TOO MUCH ALCOHOL, PHYSICAL INACTIVITY, A DIET LOW IN VITAMINS AND CALCIUM, MENOPAUSE, AND AGE

Processed meat and cancer

We know that eating lots of processed meat can increase your risk of bowel cancer. This is due to compounds, including nitrites, that are used to keep these products fresh for longer.

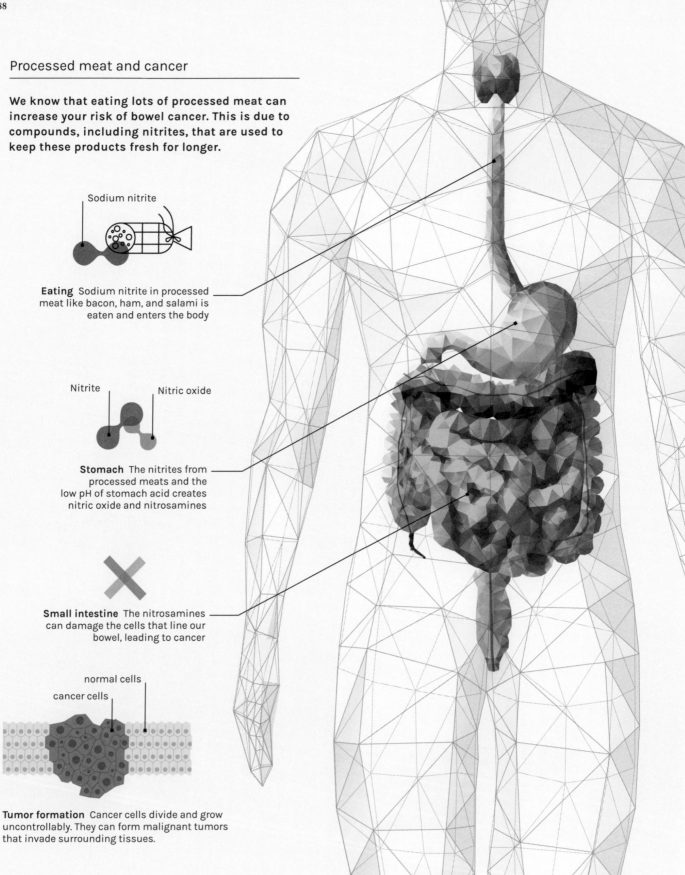

Sodium nitrite

Eating Sodium nitrite in processed meat like bacon, ham, and salami is eaten and enters the body

Nitrite   Nitric oxide

Stomach The nitrites from processed meats and the low pH of stomach acid creates nitric oxide and nitrosamines

Small intestine The nitrosamines can damage the cells that line our bowel, leading to cancer

normal cells
cancer cells

Tumor formation Cancer cells divide and grow uncontrollably. They can form malignant tumors that invade surrounding tissues.

DOES EATING A PLANT-BASED DIET PREVENT CANCER?

There are many different types of cancer—a disease caused when cells divide uncontrollably and spread into surrounding tissues. Over the years, a lot of pseudoscience has appeared regarding our diets and this disease.

There has been a great deal of research investigating the links between diet and cancer. Some foods are thought to be beneficial for some cancers and not for others, but your overall diet has a bigger impact on your cancer risk than individual foods. It's difficult to make a definitive conclusion without more research and understanding of the disease and its evolution. A lot of guidance from leading organizations around the world suggests eating a healthy balanced diet is important because some cancers are linked with body weight. Obesity is a cause of 13 different types of cancer and so eating well and maintaining a healthy body weight (see pp.204–205) is important.

Following a whole food plant-based diet may be beneficial in reducing your cancer risk as it does not contain some key dietary elements known to be a risk factor for cancer:

- **Processed and red meat**: This is known to increase the chances of colon cancer.
- **Alcohol:** Can cause seven types of cancer.
- **Foods high in calories, sugar, and fat**: Ultra-processed foods can make it harder to maintain a healthy weight.

WHOLE GRAIN AND HIGH FIBER

There is strong evidence that diets containing whole grains and fiber can protect against cancer. For total cancer mortality, studies indicate that whole grain intake is associated with a 6–12 percent lower risk of cancer when you compare those eating more whole grain versus those eating less. There was up to a 20 percent lower risk for those consuming 15–90g of fiber a day. For site-specific cancers, research has indicated that whole grain intake is consistently associated with lower risks of colon, gastric, pancreatic, and esophageal cancers. It is recommended that we eat at least 30g of fiber a day from food and include whole grains, vegetables, fruits, beans, and lentils in most meals.

DAIRY

In moderation as part of a plant-based diet, it is believed that eating and drinking milk and dairy products can reduce the risk of colon cancer.

PLANT-BASED FOR BETTER HEALTH

While there is limited research for dietary patterns such as plant-based eating or vegetarianism, recent observational studies have shown an association between reduced risk of breast cancers and bowel cancer when consuming a plant-based diet. The World Health Organization encourages a plant-based diet to increase health. Plant-based diets are an integral part of evidence-based recommendations for primary prevention of cancer and other noncommunicable diseases (NCDs), promoting a diet rich in whole grains, vegetables, fruit, nuts, and legumes and a limited consumption of red and processed meat. There's no one diet that can guarantee that you won't get cancer. But eating a healthy, balanced diet can reduce the risk.

WILL EATING PLANT-BASED PROTECT MY HEART HEALTH?

Heart disease is one of the biggest killers in the world. We know that, alongside other factors such as lack of exercise, smoking, and alcohol intake, diet can contribute to a healthy heart. Can a plant-based diet help reduce the chance of developing heart disease?

Plant-based diets can impact our heart health positively. They have been associated with a lower mortality risk compared to nonvegetarian diets and have been shown to lower heart disease risk, cholesterol, and blood pressure.

REDUCING SALT INTAKE

Salt can cause our blood pressure to rise, which, in turn, raises the risk of cardiovascular diseases such as stroke, heart failure, and heart disease. In 2017 alone, excess salt intake was linked to three million deaths globally. Around the world, people are consuming too much salt. The World Health

Organization recommends adults consume no more than 5g (2,000mg; about 1 tsp) of salt per day, yet most are reaching 8g (3,400mg) a day. Around 80 percent of the salt we consume is added to everyday items such as bread, breakfast cereals, processed meats, meat alternatives, and ready-made meals.

Plant-based diets are naturally lower in salt than those that contain meat and so switching to this way of eating will be good for your heart. Even so, remember that a lot of meat replacements, such as veggie burgers and sausages, are processed foods and have added salt and sugar to optimize taste (see pp.118–123). Try as far as possible to stick to whole

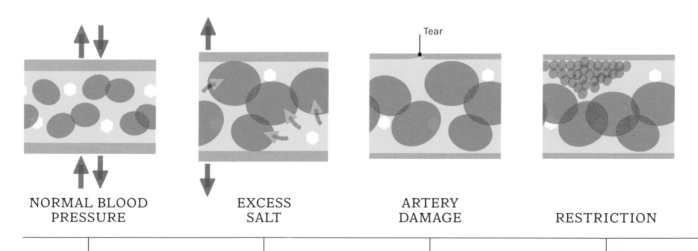

NORMAL BLOOD PRESSURE
Artery walls expand and contract as the heart pumps to circulate blood.

EXCESS SALT
The body reacts to excess salt by retaining water in the blood, increasing blood volume and pressure on arteries.

ARTERY DAMAGE
Pressure can eventually cause artery walls to narrow, tear, and stiffen, reducing blood flow.

RESTRICTION
Artery damage makes it easier for cholesterol to collect there, leading to blockages that can restrict oxygen.

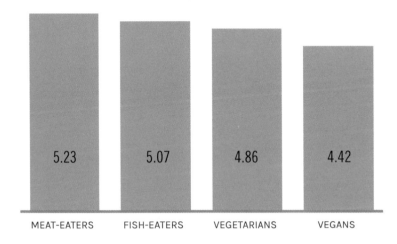

MEAT-EATERS	FISH-EATERS	VEGETARIANS	VEGANS
5.23	5.07	4.86	4.42

TOTAL CHOLESTEROL

High blood cholesterol is a factor in heart disease. The figures shown here measure blood cholesterol levels as mmol/l (millimoles per liter). Levels of cholesterol in the blood are lowest among vegans.

EAT MORE

Include these heart-healthy foods in your diet every week.

CANOLA OIL

NUTS

SEEDS

LEAFY GREEN VEGETABLES

FRUITS

EAT LESS

Avoid these foods when possible to keep your heart protected.

PROCESSED MEAT

CHIPS

WHITE BREAD

SALT

MARGARINE

foods that you prepare and cook yourself. Instead of salt, use herbs and spices for flavor because these are great additions for your gut microbiome as well as your heart.

OMEGA-3

EPA and DHA in omega-3s are especially good for your heart (see pp.102–103) as they help to reduce triglyceride levels (a type of fat in the blood), lower blood pressure, improve cholesterol profiles, and have anti-inflammatory properties.

REDUCING BLOOD PRESSURE

To keep your heart health,y you need to keep your blood pressure down. When looking to reduce blood pressure, it's recommended that you follow a plant-based diet format with a reduction in unhealthy animal-based foods, such

Salt and hypertension

High blood pressure (hypertension) in part caused by a long-term diet high in salt could potentially damage the heart, brain, and other organs.

as red and processed fatty meats and full-fat dairy foods, while adding in more nuts, seeds, vegetables, and fruit.

LOWER SATURATED FAT

A plant-based diet contains less saturated fat than one that contains animal products. Countless studies have linked the intake of dietary saturated fatty acids with an increased risk of poor heart health. Replacing the energy from saturated fat in your diet with polyunsaturated and monounsaturated fat or carbohydrate has been found to be a useful strategy for reducing the risk of heart disease. In fact, long-term trials have shown that eating less saturated fat reduces the risk of heart disease by 21 percent. Adding more olive oil, nuts, and seeds to dishes and cooking with olive, canola, or avocado oil instead of butter is a great way to increase your unsaturated fatty acid intake. In intervention studies, nuts lower total cholesterol and low-density lipoprotein (LDL) cholesterol (the cholesterol often referred to as the "bad" one), and evidence suggests that eating pulses significantly reduces LDL cholesterol levels.

DOES PLANT-BASED NUTRITION PREVENT DEMENTIA?

Dementia is the umbrella term for neurodegenerative diseases, involving loss of memory and impaired thinking that can impact everyday life. There are around 55 million people living with dementia worldwide. Scientists are working hard to see if lifestyle factors such as diet can help.

Symptoms of dementia include memory loss; confusion needing help with everyday tasks; changes in mood and behavior; and difficulties with speech, language, communication, and understanding. This happens when diseases damage the nerve cells in the brain. Different diseases damage the brain in different ways leading to different types.

The four main types of dementia are:
● Alzheimer's disease (60–70 percent of cases)
● Vascular dementia
● Dementia with Lewy bodies (closely related to Parkinson's)
● Frontotemporal dementia (FTD)

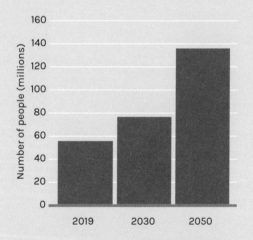

FUTURE NUMBERS OF DEMENTIA SUFFERERS

The World Health Organization predicts that the number of people with dementia is set to more than double over the next two decades.

DEMENTIA AND DIET

Dementia is currently the seventh leading cause of death and one of the major causes of disability and dependency among older people globally. Research shows that diet may help reduce this statistic. The most researched diet with top-quality studies is the Mediterranean diet, which follows plant-based diet principles. The majority of studies have shown that this way of eating is associated with improved cognitive function, a decreased risk of cognitive impairment, and a decreased risk of dementia, or Alzheimer's disease. Results from the UK biobank cohort study found that a higher Mediterranean diet adherence was associated with lower dementia risk independent of whether there was a genetic risk—this really highlights the importance of diet in risk prevention for dementia.

OMEGA-3

The latest evidence for omega-3 and brain health appears promising. One study of over 100,000 participants found good evidence that you have a reduced risk of dementia if you include omega-3 in your diet, especially in the form of DHA (see pp.102–103) and a possible 20 percent lower risk of all-cause dementia or cognitive decline. Fats from plant-based sources of omega-3 are as effective at preserving cognitive function as those from animal sources. While a healthy diet can support how our brain performs and ages, other factors such as smoking, exercise, sleep, and genetics should be considered. Diet alone cannot cure everything.

Omega-3 fatty acids and brain health

Recent studies have highlighted a link between polyunsaturated fats and brain health. They revealed that it is important to get omega-3 from different sources because different patterns of polyunsaturated fats help particular aspects of cognition by strengthening the neural circuits in the brain that can decline with age and disease.

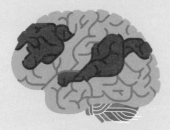

FRONTOPARIETAL CORTEX

This part of the brain is related to our ability to solve problems, reason, and adapt to new situations (fluid intelligence) and often declines more quickly than other regions of the brain, even in people without dementia.

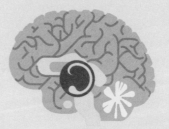

FORNIX

This group of nerve fibers at the center of the brain is important for memory and is one of the first parts of the brain to be affected by Alzheimer's disease. Omega-3 and omega-6 fatty acids can help keep the fornix healthy.

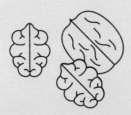

OMEGA-3 FATTY ACIDS

People with more ALA, stearidonic acid, and eicosatrienoic acid omega-3 fatty acids were found to have larger frontoparietal cortexes, which helps with fluid intelligence.

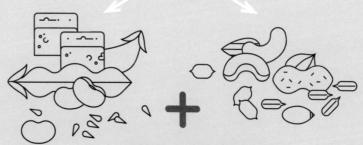

OMEGA-3 AND OMEGA-6

Research has shown that the size of the fornix is associated with a balance of omega-3 and omega-6 fatty acids in the blood. A stronger fornix is linked with memory preservation in older adults.

WILL A PLANT-BASED DIET MAKE ME LOOK YOUNGER?

Pills and potions crop up year after year with claims that they can help to ease the natural process of aging. Although you cannot physically stop aging through your diet, what you eat can impact the appearance of your skin and your overall health.

Antioxidants are often the main contributors to any research in this area, mainly vitamins A, C, and E. Eating a whole food plant-based diet provides these antioxidants, which can help prevent cellular damage and aid in removing harmful toxins from the bloodstream. Protecting the skin from one of the largest contributors of aging—sun damage—is incredibly important. Sunscreen and not exposing your skin to sun damage is the most effective way to protect your skin. The humble tomato may also help.

TOMATO POWER

Findings from a recent review suggest that foods rich in lycopene, such as tomatoes, may help the skin with sun protection. The research showed that people who ate cooked tomatoes (in large amounts) may have reduced skin erythema formation (redness of skin) and improved skin appearance and pigmentation. Lycopene may also help prevent light-induced skin photodamage and skin photo-aging. The process of cooking the tomatoes increases the bioavailability of lycopene (see pp.90–91).

SKIN AND GUT HEALTH

Many diseases of the skin are accompanied by changes in the gut microbiome, which indicates a direct link between gut health and skin. The skin is the gut's first barrier of defense against the outside environment, and what we eat may directly impact its health. Recent research has looked into the impact of diet, in particular connecting the consumption of

probiotic foods (see pp.76–77 and pp.206–207) and dermatitis, but we need more data for any conclusions to be drawn.

OLIVE OIL

Some research suggests a compound in olive oil called oleuropein may help reduce telomere shortening, which is associated with aging and has been observed during normal aging in human and in mice studies. Telomeres are nucleoprotein structures that protect the ends of DNA sequences (see above right) associated with aging.

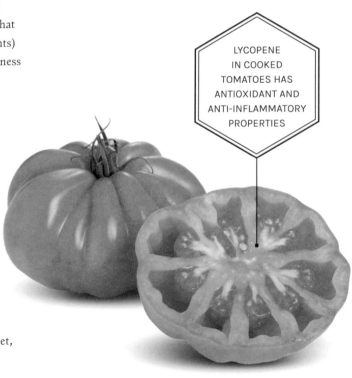

LYCOPENE IN COOKED TOMATOES HAS ANTIOXIDANT AND ANTI-INFLAMMATORY PROPERTIES

A sign of aging

Telomeres are structures at the end of DNA sequences. They prevent the ends of chromosomes from becoming frayed or tangled, which would destroy or corrupt an organism's genetic information. They shorten with age.

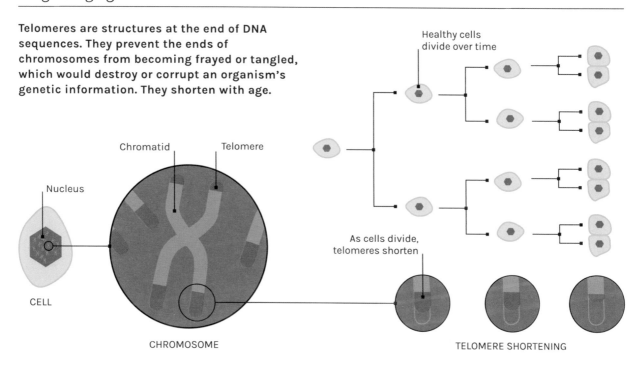

Nucleus

Chromatid

Telomere

CELL

CHROMOSOME

Healthy cells divide over time

As cells divide, telomeres shorten

TELOMERE SHORTENING

RED GRAPES

A review found evidence to suggest an agent present in red grapes and red wine, resveratrol, has been linked to anti-aging effects as it has anti-inflammatory and antioxidant properties, but this needs further research.

WATER

We often hear that water is beneficial for our skin, but there is actually very little evidence to support this. Such studies are rare, partly because water can't be patented so it is hard to find anyone to fund research when there will be no new medication or cosmetic to sell that could repay the costs. Interestingly, it may be better to sip water over a longer period of time than to drink it in one go so the body can retain more. We can measure some effect of water on the skin through the assessment of

skin turgor. This is a measure of how fast it takes the skin to return to normal if you pinch some skin and lift it up. If you are dehydrated, your skin will take longer to get its shape back.

VITAMIN C

Deficiency of vitamin C is associated with poor wound healing and fragile skin so it makes sense to include it in our diets to keep our skin healthy.

ALMONDS

Daily consumption may reduce the appearance of skin wrinkles by 16 percent and skin pigmentation in postmenopausal women. This provides evidence for a dietary contributor to reducing skin aging; however, future research should look at younger and male populations with alternative skin types to fully confirm these findings.

CAN I LOSE WEIGHT ON A PLANT-BASED DIET?

Maintaining a healthy body weight is important in order to reduce our risk of ill health. Currently, 38 percent of the world's population is obese, and this is expected to rise to 51 percent in 12 years' time, according to research by the World Obesity Federation. A good diet has never been more important.

There are many fad diets that offer unsustainable quick fixes resulting in 80–95 percent of dieters putting the weight back on when they come off a diet. Weight loss isn't as simple as energy in versus energy out; there are many factors that play a part, such as lifestyle, stress, the environment that surrounds us, sleep, genetic factors, and medication. The quality of our diet may account for more promising results with weight loss than measuring calories, which can be up to 30 percent inaccurate. We are all unique and weight loss isn't a linear process, but adopting a plant-based diet may be beneficial in helping us lose weight.

PLANT FOODS FOR WEIGHT LOSS

One review suggested plant-based diets should be considered for weight loss, with some studies using this diet alone. Others used it alongside other interventions such as fat reduction and calorie reduction. We know our gut microbes likely play a role in helping us maintain a healthy weight. Studies suggest those with more good bacteria in their guts tend to be healthier. The amount of fiber and diversity of whole foods (see pp.70–71) included within a plant-based diet may support our gut microbes and keep us full, which can help with long-term weight loss.

Waist circumference

Excess fat around the abdomen is associated with increased risk of cardiovascular disease, type 2 diabetes, and high blood pressure. You can measure your waist by holding a tape measure around your middle at the level of your navel.

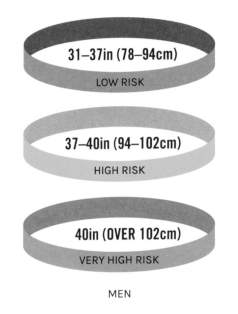

31–37in (78–94cm)
LOW RISK

37–40in (94–102cm)
HIGH RISK

40in (OVER 102cm)
VERY HIGH RISK

MEN

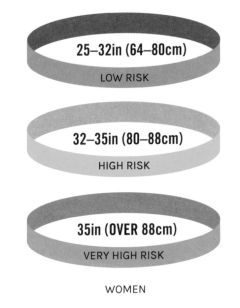

25–32in (64–80cm)
LOW RISK

32–35in (80–88cm)
HIGH RISK

35in (OVER 88cm)
VERY HIGH RISK

WOMEN

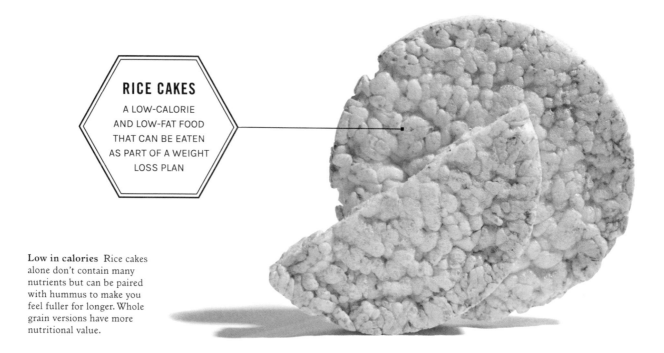

RICE CAKES

A LOW-CALORIE
AND LOW-FAT FOOD
THAT CAN BE EATEN
AS PART OF A WEIGHT
LOSS PLAN

Low in calories Rice cakes
alone don't contain many
nutrients but can be paired
with hummus to make you
feel fuller for longer. Whole
grain versions have more
nutritional value.

SOCIAL EFFECTS

Psychological and social components may help explain the success of the largely plant-based Mediterranean diet (see p.37), because societies that adopt this way of eating are very social with support mechanisms in place that are beneficial to our overall health. Psychological factors, particularly stress, trigger the release of stress hormones like cortisol. Elevated cortisol levels can influence appetite and food preferences, often leading to cravings for high-calorie, comfort foods. Hormones like leptin and ghrelin play a role in regulating hunger and fullness. Psychological factors, including stress and mental well-being, can impact the sensitivity of these hormones, affecting appetite control. Emotions and mood can influence eating behaviors as for some, consuming certain foods may activate reward pathways in the brain, which can provide a temporary sense of pleasure or comfort. This emotional eating can be influenced by social cues and environmental factors. Finally, it is clear that following a plant-based diet is beneficial for weight loss, but it has to be of good quality. It is possible to be an unhealthy plant-based eater (see pp.116–117) and not have support mechanisms and infrastructure, such as family, friends, healthy environment, and lifestyle, in place to succeed.

What works?

STICK TO A FEW TRIED-AND-TRUE PRINCIPLES TO LOSE WEIGHT AND STAY HEALTHY.

- Eat a healthy, balanced diet.
- Practice portion control.
- Eat only occasionally those less-healthy foods that you enjoy.
- Listen to your body: eat when you're hungry, and stop when you're full.
- Exercise regularly: ideally 30 minutes daily.
- Try some strategies to manage stress; it increases the hormone cortisol, which lowers blood sugar and increases food cravings.
- Get enough sleep; this will help control cortisol.

CAN I EAT A PLANT-BASED DIET IF I HAVE A FOOD INTOLERANCE?

Food intolerances are common, but some are tricky to diagnose as it's often not clear what mechanisms are causing them because, unlike allergies, they are not related to an immune system response.

INTOLERANCES

A food intolerance is when you have problems digesting certain foods. This may cause discomfort and make you feel unwell; it does not involve a reaction from the immune system. A food allergy is potentially more serious (see pp.200–201) and is caused by an abnormal attack by the body's immune system in response to eating certain proteins in foods. The most common intolerances are:

- Lactose intolerance
- Gluten intolerance
- Fructose intolerance
- Gluten sensitivity
- Food additives and natural food chemicals such as

benzoates (benzoic acid), caffeine, alcohol (ethanol), monosodium glutamate (MSG), salicylates, sulfur dioxide (sulfites), and histamines.

Celiac disease is an autoimmune response to gluten, due to high levels of an antibody that tries to attack gluten, damaging the small intestine. While gluten intolerance and celiac disease cause similar symptoms, people with gluten intolerance don't have an abnormal gene or antibodies in their blood.

SYMPTOMS

Intolerances can cause abdominal cramps, diarrhea or constipation, gas, bloating, brain fog, and aches. There are many test kits for food intolerances

---

Lactose intolerance

Lactose is a type of sugar found in most dairy products. In humans, the enzyme lactase is needed to break down lactose, so when the body doesn't produce enough lactase, the lactose passes through the gut undigested, leading to symptoms of intolerance.

KEY

- Lactase
- Lactose
- Glucose
- Galactose
- Water
- Bacteria
- Short-chain fatty acids
- Carbon dioxide
- Hydrogen
- Methane

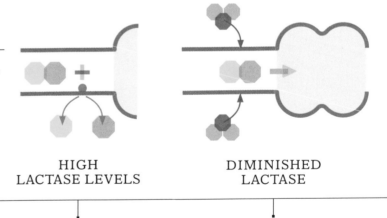

HIGH LACTASE LEVELS

Digested in small intestine
Lactase splits lactose into glucose and galactose, which can be absorbed in the blood.

DIMINISHED LACTASE

Passes small intestine
Undigested lactose moves to the large intestine and causes increased water in the colon.

available to do at home, but few are accurate. They can also be expensive, and usually, with no doctor to interpret results, they can result in unnecessary food restriction. Suspected intolerances are best diagnosed by working with your primary care physician and a specialist dietitian who will look at the following:

● Food and symptoms diary

● Elimination and reintroduction of foods to help establish triggers

● Blood tests

● Hydrogen/methane breath test (for lactose/ fructose intolerances)

PLANT-BASED DIETS AND FOOD INTOLERANCES

Fortunately, many plant-based foods such as fruits, vegetables, nuts, seeds, soy-based products, whole grains (except whole wheat, rye, and barley varieties), pulses, legumes, and beans are minimally processed and don't contain lactose, dairy, wheat, or gluten, which people are commonly intolerant to. Eating with intolerances is similar whether you're plant-based or not. Always check the labels on packaging for "may contain," "free-from," or similar claims (see pp.142–143). If a product is labeled "vegan," it may still contain traces of foods that people may be intolerant/allergic to due to unintentional cross contamination when the food is manufactured. For example, many processed plant-based meat alternatives contain wheat flour or are coated in bread crumbs.

IF FRUCTOSE OR SALICYLATE INTOLERANT?

While it is very rare, if you cannot eat fructose or salicylates and are following a plant-based diet, you will be more restricted in what you can eat as these are found in many fruits, including apples, grapes, and cherries, as well as a number of vegetables. Seek advice from your healthcare provider so that you are aware of the foods to avoid while making sure you get enough vitamins and minerals.

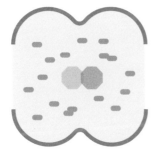

FERMENTATION

Digestion in colon
The lactose is digested by gut bacteria instead, causing fermentation.

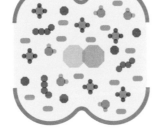

SYMPTOMS

Cramps and bloating
The increase in acids and gas caused by fermentation can lead to cramps and bloating.

ALLERGIES

MILK

FISH

CRUSTACEAN SHELLFISH

SOYBEANS

TREE NUTS

PEANUTS

SESAME

EGGS
WHEAT

INTOLERANCES

MSG

CAFFEINE

ALCOHOL

ARTIFICIAL SWEETENERS

ARTIFICIAL FOOD PRESERVATIVES

FODMAPs
(see pp.82–83)

YEAST

FRUCTOSE

LACTOSE

GLUTEN

VASO-ACTIVE AMINES
(found in red wine, strong and blue cheeses, tuna, mackerel, pork products, and other foods)

SALICYLATES

Allergies and intolerances Some foods can cause allergies while others may cause intolerances. Some foods may cause both.

CAN A PLANT-BASED DIET HELP WITH ALLERGIES?

Allergies are common, affecting up to 20 percent of populations of most developed countries. More than 100 million Americans suffer from chronic allergic diseases. Could our diets play a role in reducing these statistics?

Allergies are caused by an immune system response and can be life-threatening. Common food allergies are milk, eggs, fish, shellfish, peanuts, tree nuts, soy, and wheat. Nonfood-related allergies include pollen, dust, and mold. Allergies are often misunderstood and confused with intolerances (see pp.198–199). Understanding that they can be serious is a crucial aspect of public health nutrition to help yourself and others around you.

Food allergies affect only 2 percent of American adults and up to 4–8 percent of children. If a parent or sibling has a food allergy, the risk increases for a child to have the same. Sometimes, children outgrow these over time—this is often the case with egg allergies. If you have a food allergy, that doesn't necessarily mean your baby will, although there is a higher chance. Sadly, you can't change the biology of your body through what you eat, but diet can be used to manage the symptoms.

HAY FEVER

There is currently limited evidence that certain foods may help reduce the onset or prevent the development of hay fever, although some research suggests a diet that includes foods rich in vitamin E may be protective. Foods that contain vitamin E include almonds and avocados. Research in children has also suggested higher intakes of vitamin C, from foods such as kiwi fruits, citrus fruits, strawberries, and peppers, can help reduce hay fever symptoms too. This may be due to their antioxidant properties and their role in our immune health. However, much more scientific research and larger studies are needed to solidify these findings and understand the mechanisms behind this.

Some limited evidence from trials in Malaysia found that the daily ingestion of certain types of honey, alongside allergy medication, helped improve hay fever symptoms after four weeks. But again more research is needed to fully understand the

LEAP peanut study

A LEAP study looked at peanut allergies in children, as numbers have risen in the last 10 years. They recruited 640 babies aged 4–11 months with eczema and/or an egg allergy, as this increases the risk of having a peanut allergy. Results showed a reduced risk in babies who ate peanuts.

ATE PEANUTS
The babies who were assigned to consume peanuts had a

3.2%
chance of developing a peanut allergy

AVOIDED PEANUTS
The babies who avoided peanuts had a

17.2%
chance of developing a peanut allergy

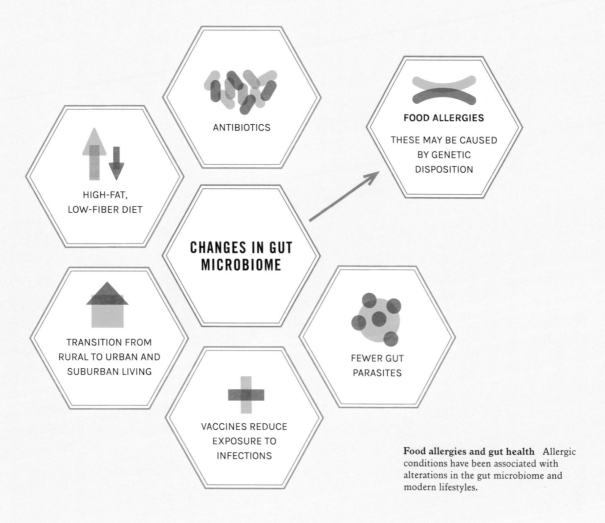

ANTIBIOTICS

FOOD ALLERGIES

THESE MAY BE CAUSED
BY GENETIC
DISPOSITION

HIGH-FAT,
LOW-FIBER DIET

CHANGES IN GUT
MICROBIOME

TRANSITION FROM
RURAL TO URBAN AND
SUBURBAN LIVING

FEWER GUT
PARASITES

VACCINES REDUCE
EXPOSURE TO
INFECTIONS

Food allergies and gut health Allergic
conditions have been associated with
alterations in the gut microbiome and
modern lifestyles.

benefits of the consumption of honey in the
prevention and/or management of hay fever. There
is also the added importance of eating local honey
and most definitely not the highly processed
varieties of honey most of us consume from
supermarkets. Infants under the age of one cannot
consume honey in any form.

Exposure to a variety of foods from conception
may prevent the development of a food allergy.
In cases where it is unavoidable and it runs in the
family or we do not know the cause, plant-based
diets cannot treat or cure an allergy, and it is best
to seek advice from a medical professional.

A RISE IN ALLERGIES?

The rise in allergies and increased sensitivity to
foods in the West are probably environmental and
related to Western lifestyles. Epidemological studies
show lower rates of allergies in developing countries.
They are also more likely to occur in urban rather
than rural areas.

Environmental factors may include increased
pollution, dietary changes, and a reduced exposure
to microbes. This is due to overuse of antibiotics or
ultra-hygiene when it comes to looking after our
homes and care of our children, which can change
how our immune systems respond to other influences.

WILL PLANT-BASED EATING CAUSE AN EATING DISORDER?

Eating disorders are complex mental health disorders that are on the rise, and more research is needed to understand the driving factors. A plant-based diet is unlikely to be the cause of an eating disorder—there will be other factors involved.

Plant-based eating can be a healthy way of life if followed flexibly, although it may contribute to the development of a potential disorder if it is used as a tool to restrict calories, fat, and ultra-processed food. Mental health issues can also be masked by healthy eating choices in some individuals. If you are concerned about an eating disorder, please seek professional medical help immediately.

THE RISE OF ORTHOREXIA

One eating disorder that is not currently fully classified is known as orthorexia, which is characterized by an obsession with healthy or "clean" eating. Sometimes a drive to live a healthy lifestyle can trigger an eating disorder and sometimes the cause is unknown. Over the past few years, clinicians working with patients with eating disorders have noted a rise in the number of patients reporting to be vegan, although there is limited research in this area. During eating disorder treatment, some people will report that they became pescatarian, vegetarian, or vegan. However, these socially acceptable restrictions may mask the development of an eating disorder—and therefore may be a part of their illness.

VEGETARIANISM AND ANOREXIA

Vegetarianism is more researched than veganism, and research from 2015 found 34.8 percent of patients in treatment for an eating disorder were vegetarian, while vegetarians made up 6.8 percent of those with no disordered eating history. In those seeking help for anorexia nervosa, over half were practicing a vegetarian diet. Studies also found that people with an eating disorder following a vegetarian diet reported eating disorder symptoms before choosing to be vegetarian, with an average of one year between the development of eating disorder symptoms and becoming vegetarian. So it seems as though vegetarianism can sometimes mask anorexia and other eating disorders as it is perceived as being both socially and environmentally friendly, which means it is less likely to raise concerns in others.

Generally speaking, any form of dietary restriction has the potential to contribute to the development of an eating disorder. However, the research that has been done in this area seems to suggest that if people become vegan or vegetarian for ethical reasons, rather than to change their physical appearance, then they are less likely to develop problems of this nature.

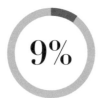

9% EATING DISORDERS AFFECT AT LEAST 9% OF THE POPULATION WORLDWIDE

LESS THAN 6% OF PEOPLE WITH EATING DISORDERS ARE MEDICALLY DIAGNOSED AS "UNDERWEIGHT"

ONE DEATH EVERY 52 MINUTES IS THE DIRECT RESULT OF AN EATING DISORDER

Recovery goals

The Recovery from Eating Disorders for Life (REAL) Food Guide was produced in 2018 to support recovery goals for those experiencing eating disorders. It recognizes that recovery from eating disorders requires emphasis on choosing a variety of foods, including energy-dense foods. This vegan version of the pyramid has been created to ensure support is provided for those on a plant-based diet.

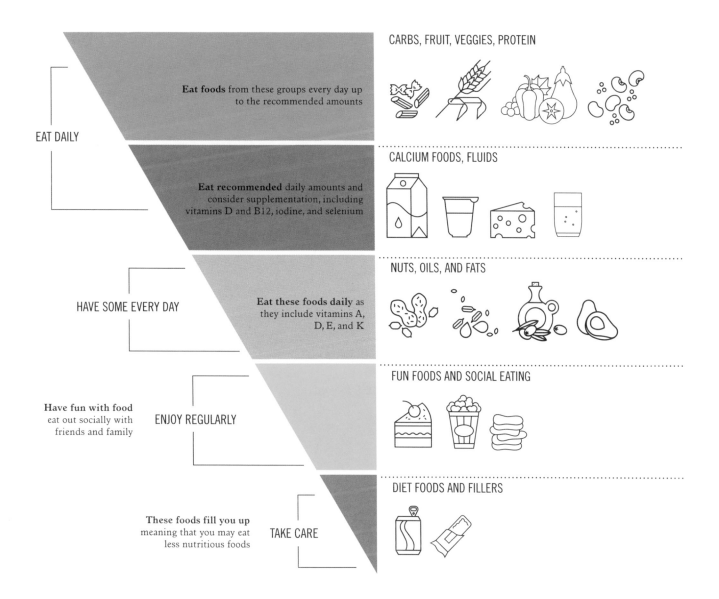

EAT DAILY

Eat foods from these groups every day up to the recommended amounts

CARBS, FRUIT, VEGGIES, PROTEIN

Eat recommended daily amounts and consider supplementation, including vitamins D and B12, iodine, and selenium

CALCIUM FOODS, FLUIDS

HAVE SOME EVERY DAY

Eat these foods daily as they include vitamins A, D, E, and K

NUTS, OILS, AND FATS

Have fun with food eat out socially with friends and family

ENJOY REGULARLY

FUN FOODS AND SOCIAL EATING

These foods fill you up meaning that you may eat less nutritious foods

TAKE CARE

DIET FOODS AND FILLERS

WILL A PLANT-BASED DIET HELP WITH OBESITY?

Worldwide, obesity has nearly tripled since 1975. There are many different reasons for this, including the environment we live in; inactive lifestyles; education around food; the proliferation of energy-dense foods high in fat, sugars, and salt; and genetics. Will eating more plant foods help?

Obesity is defined by abnormal or excessive fat accumulation that may impair health. It isn't a lifestyle choice and is often misunderstood. Psychological factors and individual relationships with food that can cause people to overeat are often overlooked. A lack of support that can help us make healthy changes is a key area of concern—dietary and physical lifestyle changes often involve a lot of thought and planning. Outside support, including societal changes and policies in sectors such as the urban planning environment, can affect weight management. For example, if we build new homes and plan urban areas that are designed around walking or cycling to a destination instead of using cars for short trips, that may help improve obesity levels over the long term.

FIBER INTAKE

Plant-based diets, if executed well, could help many on their journey to a healthier body and body fat loss. Plant-based diets typically contain high amounts of fiber from whole foods, plants, beans, and pulses, which is associated with lower long-term weight gain. As we consume more dietary fiber, we are likely to reduce our overall energy intake as we feel full and satisfied after eating. When we eat more high-energy foods (often processed foods containing high levels of salt, sugar, and fat), we can often feel unsatisfied and eat more, leading to obesity. Higher levels of fiber in the gut slows the absorption of cholesterol and causes changes in the gut microbiota, producing short-chain fatty acids (see pp.16–17), which can help regulate appetite,

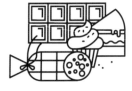

Eating mindfully

Weight loss in the long term depends on healthy habits that we can maintain. Eating mindfully means making sensible decisions and considering your eating habits, which can help you avoid poor choices and weight gain.

ELIMINATE DISTRACTIONS

Leave your phone and laptop in another room and try to stop and savor your food, even if only for a short amount of time.

PORTION CONTROL

Try to eat when you're hungry and stop when you're satisfied. Avoid processed foods and stick to sensible portion sizes.

reduce abdominal fat, and improve insulin sensitivity, thereby reducing the likelihood of developing type 2 diabetes.

WEIGHT-LOSS STUDIES

Studies have shown diets higher in plants and lower in animal products resulted in increased weight loss over a six-month period. The type of diet varies between individuals and is difficult to measure, but simple switches like reducing meat and adding pulses may be helpful. One study assigned participants to either a vegan, vegetarian, pescatarian, semi-vegetarian, or omnivorous diet, along with recipe guidance, glycemic index (GI) information, and dietitian advice. All the groups lost a significant amount of weight after two months and six months, compared with their starting weight. Weight loss was, however, greatest in the vegan group, which indicates that eating more plants and less animal produce may be a useful tool in weight loss.

DIABETES

Risk of type 2 diabetes has been found to be reduced when following a plant-based diet. As type 2 diabetes and obesity are linked, this suggests that following a plant-based diet may reduce obesity risk. The DASH diet (Dietary Approaches to Stop Hypertension), which includes whole foods, fruit, vegetables, beans, and small amounts of animal products has been linked with improved regulation of blood sugar levels, which is associated with reduced obesity risk. The Mediterranean diet (see p.37) has been found to reduce risk of type 2 diabetes.

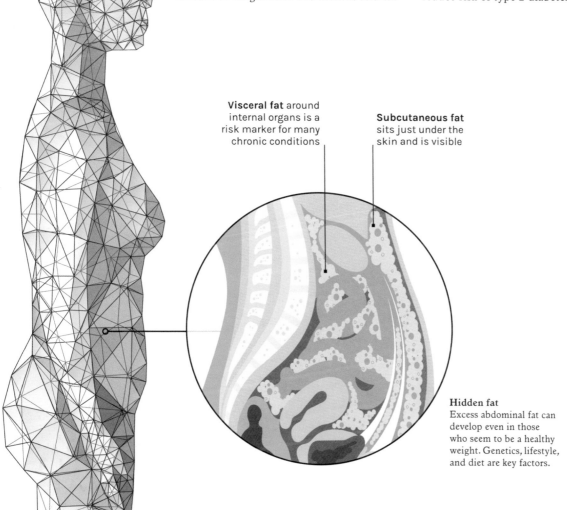

Visceral fat around internal organs is a risk marker for many chronic conditions

Subcutaneous fat sits just under the skin and is visible

Hidden fat
Excess abdominal fat can develop even in those who seem to be a healthy weight. Genetics, lifestyle, and diet are key factors.

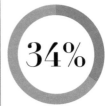

IN 2016, MORE THAN

1.9 BILLION

ADULTS AGED 18 YEARS AND OLDER, WERE OVERWEIGHT

34%

OF THESE—OVER 650 MILLION—WERE OBESE

39 MILLION

CHILDREN UNDER THE AGE OF 5 WERE OVERWEIGHT OR OBESE IN 2020

HOW DOES PLANT-BASED EATING AFFECT OUR SKIN AND MOUTH?

While there is now increasing research into gut health, the impact that diet can have on the oral and skin microbiomes is less understood. So what do we know so far? Can what we eat positively impact our skin and mouth microbiomes?

THE SKIN MICROBIOME

The skin's microbiome is often referred to as the skin flora. There are around 1,000 diverse microorganisms that live on human skin. Most are found in the superficial layers of the epidermis and the upper parts of hair follicles. A balance between these different microorganisms helps maintain skin health and prevent harmful pathogens from developing. The skin microbiome also provides protection against harmful microorganisms and helps modulate the immune system.

There has been some research into individual micronutrient deficiencies and skin, but there is limited evidence from clinical studies for specific foods or diets. A higher consumption of foods commonly included in plant-based diets showed less skin damage caused by persistent sun exposure compared to foods in a typical Western diet such as full-fat milk, red and processed meat, potatoes, sugar-sweetened drinks, cakes, and pastries.

We have some further data that addresses the effects of plant-based versus Western diets on skin health and how these diets interact with the gut microbiome and the effect they have on overall skin health. Western diets have been shown to negatively impact skin health by causing a disruption to and dysregulation of the gut microbiome, which, in turn, may lead to issues with skin health, such as decreased elasticity, firmness, and depigmentation. Conversely, plant-based diets have been associated with healthier skin because they enrich, improve, and modulate the gut microbiome.

THE ORAL MICROBIOME

The oral microbiome is the second-most diverse and plentiful microbiota in the human body after the gut. While there have been studies looking at the effect of diet on inflammation or infection of the gums and bones surrounding the teeth and how this impacts the oral microbiome, there has not been as much research on the effect of diet on the microorganisms that inhabit the oral cavity.

The health of the oral microbiome varies depending on our age, our mother's microbiota, which can be passed on, and factors such as how you clean your teeth, whether or not you smoke, genetics, and your general health.

Some studies suggest the diet we consume and the subsequent oral microbiome may be directly linked to obesity (although the reasons for this are unclear). The oral microbiome may also affect cardiovascular health (related to inflammation), and insulin resistance (thought to be related to inflammation that affects the entire body). Another study of 78 vegans and 82 omnivores observed that the oral microbiota of vegans differed significantly from that of omnivores. More research is needed to confirm the associations and the longer-term impacts of plant-based eating and specific nutrients or components of plant-based eating on the oral microbiome.

Generally, if you aim for a diverse diet that does not leave you deficient in nutrients, don't overconsume sugar and alcohol, and live a healthy lifestyle, your oral microbiome will be healthier.

Eating for your skin

Western diets have been shown to negatively impact skin health by causing a disruption of our gut microbiome. This can lead to decreased skin elasticity and pigmentation.

A balanced and diverse oral microbiome is needed for good oral health

WESTERN DIET
DYSREGULATION OF MICROBIOTA

Microbiome composition Higher levels of processed foods and less fiber reduces microbiobal diversity

REDUCED
ELASTICITY
FIRMNESS
PIGMENTATION

PLANT-BASED DIET
IMPROVEMENT IN MICROBIOTA DUE TO INCREASED AND VARIED FIBER INTAKE

More fiber and whole foods in a plant-based diet leads to more short-chain fatty acids (see p.69), which improves our skin microbiome

INCREASED
ELASTICITY
FIRMNESS
PIGMENTATION

NUTRITION TABLES

These tables show the recommended intake of key nutrients at different ages.
It is important to be aware of these when eating a plant-based diet.

PROTEIN

AGE	RDA* (G PER DAY)
0–6 months	12.5–12.7
7–12 months	13.7–14.9
1–9 years	14.5–19
7–10 years	28.3
11–14 years	41.2 (female), 42.1 (male)
15–18 years	45.4 (female), 55.2 (male)
18 years +	0.8 per kg (2.2lb) body weight
Breastfeeding/lactation (in addition to the female requirements of 0.8g per kg/2.2lb body weight per day)	+11g when baby is 0–6 months +8g when baby is 6 months+

When 18 years and above, the Recommended Daily
Allowance (RDA) is set at 0.8g of protein per
kilogram (2.2lb) body weight per day for adults. For
example: If an adult weighs 60kg (132lb), they would
require 60 x 0.8 = 48g protein per day. However, it is
important to note that if you are very active, you
may require more protein than the average person.

IRON

AGE	RDA* (MG PER DAY)
0–6 months	0.27
7–12 months	11
1–3 years	7
4–8 years	10
9–13 years	8
14–18 years	11 (male), 15 (female)
19–50 years	8 (male), 18 (female)
51 years +	8
Pregnant women	27

ZINC

AGE	RDA* (MG PER DAY)
0–6 months	2
7–12 months	3
1–3 years	3
4–8 years	5
9–13 years	8
14–18 years	11 (male), 9 (female)
19 years +	11 (male), 8 (female)
Breastfeeding	12

FIBER

AGE	RDA* (G PER DAY)
2–5 years	15
5–12 years	20
11–16 years	25
17 + years	30

OMEGA-3

The Dietary Guidelines for Americans 2015–2020
recommends 450–500mg of omega-3 fatty acids per
day. Those with coronary heart disease should
consume 1g of omega-3 fatty acid per day, preferably
from fatty fish.

IODINE

AGE	RDA* (MCG PER DAY)	WHO** (MCG PER DAY)
0-6 months	110	90
7-12 months	130	90
1-3 years	90	90
4-8 years	90	120
9-13 years	120	120
14-18 years	150	150
19 years +	150	150
Breastfeeding	290 (pregnancy: 220)	250 (pregnancy: 250)

CALCIUM

AGE	RDA* (MG PER DAY)
0-6 months	200
7-12 months	260
1-3 years	700
4-8 years	1,000
9-13 years	1,300
14-18 years	1,300
19-50 years	1,000
50+ years	1,200

CALCIUM ABSORBABILITY	RDA* (MG PER DAY)
Good (around 30-50%)	Fortified plant-based dairy alternative drinks, calcium-set tofu, low oxalate vegetables such as kale, broccoli, Brussels sprouts, bok choy, watercress, spring greens
Fair (around 20%)	Pinto beans, red beans, white beans
Poor (around 10% or less)	Sesame seeds, rhubarb
Very poor (around 5%)	Spinach

*RDA = Recommended Daily Allowance. The average daily level of intake needed to meet the nutrient requirements of healthy individuals.

**WHO = World Health Organization

The tables on these pages compare the best sources of those same nutrients. These are plant-based where possible but include meat, fish, and dairy sources where plants alone can't supply without supplementation.

FOOD		PROTEIN (PER 100G)
Pulses	Red lentils, canned	7.5g
	Chickpeas, canned	7.2g
	Peas, frozen or boiled	6g
Tofu	Tofu	6g
Beans	Red kidney beans	6.9g
	Black-eyes peas	8.8g
	Baked beans	5.2g
Quorn	Quorn	9g
TVP	Soy crumbles	17g
Nuts	Peanut butter	22.6g
	Almonds	21.1g
	Cashews	20.5g
	Walnuts	14.7g
	Hazelnuts	14.1g
	Brazil nuts	14.1g
	Pistachios	17.9g
	Pecans	9.2g
	Macadamia nuts	7.9g
Seeds	Chia seeds	18g
	Hemp seeds	35g
	Sesame seeds	18.2g
	Sunflower seeds	19.8g
	Pumpkin seeds	24.4g
Grains	Basmati rice	2.6g
	Quinoa	4.7g
	Oats	1.4g
	Whole wheat bread	9.4g
	Barley	2.7g

FOOD		IRON (PER 100G)
Legumes (cooked)	Red lentils	2.3mg
	Green lentils	3.5mg
	Puy lentils	3.5mg
	Chickpeas	2mg
	Black beans	2.1mg
	Lima beans	1.5mg
	Kidney beans	2mg
	Falafel	3.4mg
	Hummus	1.9mg
Grains (uncooked)	Rolled oats	3.6mg
	Quinoa	7.8mg
	Pasta	1.8mg
	Lentil pasta	7.6mg
Green leafy vegetables	Broccoli, steamed	1mg
	Spinach, boiled	1.6mg
Fortified cereals	Fortified wheat-based cereal	11.9mg

FOOD	PORTION SIZE	ZINC
Quorn	100g	7mg
Tofu, steamed	75g	1.5mg
Sun-dried tomatoes in oil	35g	0.3mg
Chickpeas	1100g	0.8mg
Red kidney beans	100g	0.7mg
Red lentils	100g	1mg
Green/brown lentils	100g	1.4mg
Soybeans	100g	0.9mg
Cashew nuts	30g	1.7mg
Brazil nuts	30g	1.3mg
Almonds	30g	1mg
Pecans	30g	1.6mg
Peanuts	30g	1.1mg
Peanut butter	40g	1.2mg
Tahini paste	19g	1mg
Hummus	60g	0.8mg
Hemp seeds	10g	1mg
Pumpkin seeds	10g	0.7mg
Flaxseeds	10g	0.5mg
Chia seeds	10g	0.4mg
Sesame seeds	7g	0.4mg

FOOD	PORTION SIZE	IODINE
Cow's milk	100ml	25–50mcg
Yogurt	75g	25–50mcg
Fortified dairy alternative drink	100ml	13–30mcg
Eggs	1 egg	25mcg
Cod	60g	115mcg
Salmon	50g	7mcg
Haddock	60g	195mcg
Canned tuna	50g	6mcg
Shrimp	30g	3mcg
Scampi	85g	80mcg
Nori sheets	1 sheet	42mcg

FOOD		PORTION SIZE	CALCIUM
Dairy products	Breast milk	100ml	30–40mg
	Milk (all other types)	200ml	240mg
	Yogurt	45g	60mg
	Cheese	Around 30g	120mg
Calcium-fortified nondairy products	Fortified dairy milk alternatives (Soy/pea/oat/nut drinks)	200ml	240mg
	Fortified dairy alternative yogurts (e.g. soy)	125g	150mg
	Fortified dairy alternative Cheddar-type cheese	15g	120mg
	Soybean curd/tofu (only if set with calcium chloride or calcium sulfate)	60g	200mg
	Fortified dairy alternative Cheddar-type cheese	15g	120mg
	Calcium-fortified infant cereals	1 serving	60–120mg
	Calcium-fortified cereals	30g	130–150g
	Calcium-fortified bread	1 slice (around 40g)	191mg
Nondairy products	Sardines (with bones)	60g	258mg
	Whitebait	50g	430mg
	Broccoli, boiled	85g	34mg
	Kale, boiled	20g	30mg
	Okra, boiled	25g	30mg
	Bok choy	30g	30mg
	Sesame seeds	1 tsp	27mg
	Tahini	1 tsp	40mg
	Sesame seeds	1 tsp	27mg
	Almonds, ground	1 tbsp	17mg

FOOD	PORTION SIZE	FIBER
Red kidney beans	3 tbsp	4g
Raspberries	10 raspberries	2.7g
Avocado	1/4 of an avocado	2g
Chickpeas	3 tbsp	2g
Oats (dry)	25g	2g
Red lentils	3 tbsp	2g
Carrot	1/2 carrot	2g
Apple	1/2 apple	1g
Chia seeds	1 tsp	1.2g
Hummus	2 tbsp	2.5g

FOOD		OMEGA-3 (PER 100G)		
		SFA (G)	MUFA (G)	PUFA (G)
Nuts	Almonds	3.8	31.6	12.4
	Cashews	17.4	22.4	25.4
	Brazil Nuts	9.5	27.8	8.8
	Hazelnuts	4.6	49.2	6.6
	Macadamia nuts	11.2	60.8	1.6
	Peanuts	8.7	22	13.1
	Pecans	5.7	42.5	18.7
	Pistachios	7.4	27.6	17.9
	Walnuts	7.5	10.7	46.8
Seeds	Chia	3.2	2.2	27.4
	Hemp	4.7	5.6	36.8
	Flaxseed	4.1	7.7	12.1
	Pumpkin	7	11.2	18.3
	Sunflower	4.5	9.8	31
	Sesame	8.3	21.7	25.5
Fruit	Avocado	4.1	12.1	2.2
	Coconut milk	16.6	1.2	0.3

SFA = Saturated fatty acids

MUFA = Monounsaturated fatty acids

PUFA = Polyunsaturated fatty acids

INDEX

iodine 108–109
  plant-based diets and **160–61**
  vitamin B12 111
premenstrual syndrome (PMS) **170–71**
pressure cookers **156–57**
probiotics **76–77**, 89, 178, **185**
processed food 21, 32, 94, 190
  definition of **60, 61**
  gut bacteria and 17
  meat 51, 58, **188**, 189, 191
  obesity and 204
  plant-based **60–61**
  reducing consumption of **178**
proline 165
propionate 69, 78
prostaglandins 171
prostate cancer 180
protease inhibitors 91
protein 10, 15, **20–21**, 27, 29, 86, **92–93**
  complete proteins **92**
  plant-based athletes 174–75
  portion sizes 26
  protein synthesis 99
  recommended intake **92, 164**
  sources of 52, **54**, 56, **92–93**, **129**, **131**, 183
proteins 14
pseudograins **132**
public health nutritional guidelines 10
pulses 48, 70, **71**, 81, 131
pyridoxine **23**, 55, 58, 91, 143, 185

Q

quinoa 21, 92, 93, 132
Quorn *see* mycoprotein

R

Recommended Dietary Intake (RDI) **86**
Recovery from Eating Disorders for Life (REAL)
  Food Guide **203**
rectum **12**, 13, 16, 89
red blood cells 22, 23, 98, 110, 136, 164
red kidney beans 80, 92, **130**, 131
reflux disease 16
reproductive system 106
respiratory illnesses 29, 77
resveratrol 67, 68, 79, 195
riboflavin **22**, 55, 58, 91, 124
rice 26, 27, 42, 78
rice cakes 197
rice milk **135**
rickets 29, 166
roasting 152

S

salads 72, 73
salicylate 199
saliva 12, 88
salmon 52, 53
salt 28, 30, 31, 32, 46, 47, 61
  daily maximum 142
  and hypertension **190–91**
  reducing **190–91**
saponins **127**
sardines 52
satiation 27
saturated fat **21**, 28, 31, 32, **33**, 44, 47, 51,
  62, 63, **191**
  coconut 146, 147
sauerkraut 78
scurvy, preventing **11**
seaweed 108, 109, **136–37**, 148
sedentary lifestyles 18
seeds 26, 27, 48, 63, 70, **71**, 73
seitan 92, **120–21**, 149

selenium **23**, 46, 67, 86, **106–107**
  deficiency **106–107**
  soil and **107**
  sources of 32, 55, 58, 91
  supplements 96
  why you need it **107**
selenoproteins 106
serotonin 68, 177, **178**, **179**
short-chain fatty acids (SCFAs) 66, **69**,
  70, 74, 78, 185, 204–205
skin health 22, 23, 66
  aging **182–83**
  and almonds **195**
  benefits of good nutrition **29**, 207
  benefits of hydration 25
  and fiber 207
  and gut health **194**, 206, 207
  looking younger **194–95**
  olive oil and **194**
  plant-based diets and **206–207**
  skin microbiome **206**
  tomatoes and **194**
  and vitamin C **195**
  water and **195**
  zinc as treatment for 112, **113**
skins, fruit and vegetable 49, 153
sleep 17, 18, 69, 184, 197
  plant-based diets and **176–77**
slow cookers 153
small intestine **12**, 13, 16, 81, 83, 89, 198
smoothies 73
snacks 49, 60
sodium **23**
sodium nitrate 188
soil 108, 144
soups 73
sourdough 78
soy sauce 148–49
soy 21, 92, **130**, 176
  and menopause **118**, 119, 168, 169
  servings **119**

ACKNOWLEDGMENTS

BIBLIOGRAPHY

To access a full list of research citations supporting the information in this book, please visit:

https://www.dk.com/us/information/science-of-plant-based-nutrition-biblio/

AUTHOR'S ACKNOWLEDGMENTS

This book has been more than just a project fueled by passion; it is my genuine hope that it serves as a meaningful contribution toward the positive cause of preserving our planet.

This endeavor is a collective mission, made possible by the invaluable contributions of numerous individuals without whom this would not have been achievable. The exceptional DK team, including Nicola, Alastair, and Cara, alongside the design prowess of Amy and Sarah, and the captivating photography by Nigel and Sun's team, all embody extraordinary talent and dedication, crucial in bringing this book to fruition.

My fantastic team of researchers and nutrition students—Amy Woods, Beth Tripp, Olivia Rosenvinge, Aoibhínn Connolly—deserve special mention for their invaluable contributions. I must express particular gratitude to my right-hand women, Eleanor Morris and Abi Robertson. Observing the genuine pleasure they've experienced while immersing themselves in the latest scientific research has been truly heartening.

My outstanding Rhitrition clinic team, including Sarah Elder, Mala Watts, Lisa Waldron, Faye Townsend, Catherine Rabess, the meticulous proofreader and peer reviewer. Their efforts have ensured this book is the best version it can possibly be. A special recognition goes to Meg and Dola for their crucial help every step of the way. Balancing the demands of motherhood and business ownership is a significant challenge, and I consider myself truly fortunate to be surrounded by such an exceptional team.

Finally, I must acknowledge my family. My two boys, Zachary and Theodore, serve as constant inspiration, motivating me to contribute positively to the world. I'm grateful to my dad for his attentive ear, and to my husband, Billy, as his understanding, patience, and unwavering support through both the highs and lows make me feel like the luckiest person in the world.

PUBLISHER'S ACKNOWLEDGMENTS

Dorling Kindersley would like to thank Vanessa Bird for indexing; Kathy Steer for proofreading; Ginger Hultin for consulting on the US edition; Nigel Wright/XAB Design for photographic styling; and Lucy-Ruth Hathaway for food styling.

PICTURE CREDITS

The publisher would like to thank the following for their kind permission to reproduce their photographs:

(Key: a-above; b-below/bottom; c-centre; f-far; l-left; r-right; t-top)

7 123RF.com: Annarosa84. **91 Dreamstime.com:** Draftmode. **117 Dreamstime.com:** Anny Ben (c); Saletomic (cla). **121 Dreamstime.com:** Picture Partners. **124 Dreamstime.com:** Mona Makela. **133 Dreamstime.com:** Ekaterina Kriminskaia. **136 Dreamstime.com:** Harutora. **203** Diagram adapted from work by Lisa Waldron

All other images © Dorling Kindersley

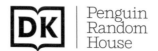

DK LONDON

Editorial Director Cara Armstrong
Senior Editor Alastair Laing
US Senior Editor Jennette ElNaggar
Senior Designer Sarah Snelling
Production Editor David Almond
Production Controller Kariss Ainsworth
Jacket Coordinator Emily Cannings
Jacket Designer Izzy Poulson
Art Director Maxine Pedliham
Publishing Director Katie Cowan

Editorial Nicola Hodgson
Design Amy Child
Illustration Sally Caulwell, Nelli Velichko
Photography Sun Lee, Stephanie McLeod

First American Edition, 2024
Published in the United States by DK Publishing,
a division of Penguin Random House LLC
1745 Broadway, 20th Floor, New York, NY 10019

A catalog record for this book
is available from the Library of Congress.
ISBN 978-0-7440-9910-2

Printed and bound in China

www.dk.com

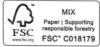

This book was made with Forest
Stewardship Council™ certified
paper—one small step in DK's
commitment to a sustainable future.
Learn more at **www.dk.com/uk/
information/sustainability**

ABOUT THE AUTHOR

Rhiannon Lambert is one of the UK's leading nutritionists, a bestselling author, and chart-topping podcast host.

In 2016, she founded Rhitrition, a renowned Harley Street clinic, which specializes in weight management, sports nutrition, eating disorders, and pre- and postnatal nutrition. Its highly qualified, professional team of registered nutritionists, registered dietitians, and chartered psychologists work with individuals to transform their lives.

As an evidence-based practitioner, Rhiannon is committed to the benefits of a scientific approach to nutrition.

She has worked as a consultant to many well-known food brands, refining their menus, product ranges, and cooking methodology. Rhiannon has also advised on nutrition and well-being at some of the world's exclusive hospitality destinations.

In 2017, Rhiannon published her first book, the bestselling *Re-Nourish: A Simple Way to Eat Well,* part handbook, part cookbook, in which she shares her food philosophy to lay the foundations for a happy, healthy relationship with eating. She followed this up in 2019 with *Top of Your Game: Eating for Mind & Body*, co-written with world snooker champion, Ronnie O'Sullivan. In 2021, she wrote the first book in this series, *The Science of Nutrition: Debunk the Diet Myths and Learn How to Eat Well for Health and Happiness.* In 2022, she published *Deliciously Healthy Pregnancy: Nutrition and Recipes for Optimal Health from Conception to Parenthood.*

Rhiannon also has her own food supplements company, Rhitrition+. A healthy, balanced diet should provide all the nutrients your body needs, but, sometimes, for all sorts of reasons, it falls short. Rhitrition+'s innovative approach uses Rhiannon's evidence-based, scientifically sound formulas to produce supplements for the vitamins and minerals lacking in many diets.

Rhiannon hosts the top-rated "Food for Thought" podcast, which gives listeners practical, evidence-based advice on how to achieve a healthier lifestyle. With more than seven million downloads since 2018, it is firmly established as one of the UK's most popular health podcasts.

Registered with the Association for Nutrition, Rhiannon obtained a first-class degree in Nutrition and Health; a master's degree in Obesity, Risks, and Prevention; and diplomas in sports nutrition and in pre- and postnatal nutrition. She is a Master Practitioner in Eating Disorders, accredited by The British Psychological Society, and a Level 3 Personal Trainer.

Follow Rhiannon on Instagram, TikTok, Twitter, Facebook, and YouTube at @Rhitrition and visit Rhitrition.com